A Country Chemist

Memoirs of a Rural Pharmacist

by

Rex Merchant

A Country Chemist
Memoirs of a Rural Pharmacist

by

Rex Merchant

Published by

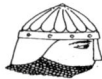

Rex Merchant
@ Norman Cottage

Published by
Rex Merchant @ Norman Cottage
89 West Rd. Oakham. Rutland. LE15 6LT
normancottage@ yahoo.co.uk
www.rexmerchant.co.uk

British Library Cataloguing- in - Publication Data.
A catalogue record of this book is available from the
British Library

Cover designed, text typeset, printed and bound by
Rex Merchant @ Norman Cottage.

INDEX

Author's Notes

I qualified as a Pharmacist in 1958 and worked in retail pharmacy for over 40 years; I started an apprenticeship in 1953 and retired in 1995. I was a store manager for the Boots Company and a Graduate Tutor for trainee pharmacists. During my retail career I have seen and experienced many profound changes in my chosen profession.

I worked in rural pharmacies prefering the pace and the friendliness of a country environment. The chance to really get to know the customers and to make a difference to their lives was more important than promotion to a city business. I much preferred the country environment for my family.

My two daughters were born when I lived and worked at Uppingham. They enjoyed a safe country upbringing and an excellent schooling in Rutland. Both went on to DeMontfort University to earn BA Degrees.

Rural pharmacy brings its own rewards and problems. Business is tied to the seasons and the farming community as well as the medical needs of the local inhabitants. Living in a rural area also effects one's opportunities for hobbies and after work activities; I have written about some of my own interests to give a rounded view of my life as a rural pharmacist.

I have enjoyed my time in the pharmacy profession and have tried to give a flavour of my daily life as a rural chemist.

Rex Merchant   M.R.Pharm.S.
Oakham.   2015

Chapter One - The Journey Begins

When I left Spalding Grammar School in 1953, I had already decided I wanted to study to become a Pharmacist. I've no idea why I fancied that profession, I knew no one who already practised it and had never been behind the scenes at a dispensary, but my favourite subject was Chemistry, closely followed by Physics and Maths, so I can only assume I thought being a Chemist would best suit my interests. It was a haphazard way to pick a future career but it proved to be a happy choice. In those days at Grammar School, unless you wanted to be a teacher or a doctor, there was no careers advice offered.

I left school before the end of term, immediately after the exams were over, and went to work on the land to earn some money. My mother was bringing up myself and my young sister on her own by doing land work, so she badly needed the help. I applied to Boots the Chemist in Spalding for a place as an apprentice. In those days pharmacy students served a two year indentured apprenticeship before doing their three year pharmacy course. There was no vacancy at Spalding, my home town, but a place was eventually found for me at Holbeach, which was eight miles from my home.

When I first left school and worked on the land I worked from 8am to 8pm and at weekends, earning a very good wage. I had the opportunity to use my schooboy French when I ran a bulb company's prepacking department, which was staffed with French exchange students. Some weeks I took home as much as £15, which was the same as my first salary some five years later as a qualified chemist! When I started in the November at Boots store in Holbeach, my income dropped dramatically. I earned 35 shillings (£1-75p) a week with an aditional allowance of 8 shillings (40p) a week to cover my bus fares. In fine weather I always cycled the sixteen mile round trip to work and back to save spending the bus fares, but in winter I was forced to use the bus.

There was one big problem with the Holbeach bus service; it left Spalding rather early and got me into Holbeach at just after 8am, three quarters of an hour before the Boots manager turned up to open the store. This was particularly inconvenient in the depths of winter; waiting outside all that time in the cold was no pleasure. Next door to the Boots store was a baker. After a few freezing cold episodes standing outside the Boots store on the pavement waiting for the manager to open the shop, the baker took pity on me and invited me into his bakehouse, which was behind his confectioner's shop. This arrangement was perfect; it was warm because he had been using his oven from early morning. I sat all snug and warm talking to the elderly baker and listening to the chirping Crickets, which also inhabited that warm room. I used to treat myself to a newly made cream cake most mornings to eat with my cup of tea at break time.

Holbeach Boots was a small pharmacy in a fenland village. The business was mainly Farms and Gardens with a heavy bias towards horticulture as the village was in the centre of the South Holland, fenland growing area. Local farmers grew flowers such as Tulips, Daffodils, Narcissi and Gladioli. They grew food crops in the fields such as Peas, Beans, Potatoes, Cereals, Sugar Beet and crops under glass such as Tomatoes. There were a few sheep and cattle kept on some of the fields out on the marsh near the sea banks but most of the land was far too productive to be put down to grass. When I joined the staff at Holbeach I was employed in the Farms and Gardens department and saw nothing of the dispensary. My boss, George Toplis, did not give me the opportunity to learn the pharmacy side of the business but kept me busy where he made most of his money, on the farming side.

Boots supplied a correspondence course to their pharmacy apprentices. I spent one afternoon a week studying this course in the staff room. I was also expected to complete the course they used to train their farms and gardens staff. The modern post-graduate pharmacy students have to pass an exam at the end of their year of practical traning before they can register to practise their profession. There was no such examination in the 1950s so there was little check on the standard of the training given.

After three quarters of my time had passed as an apprentice, George Toplis was promoted to the larger Boots store at Saffron Walden and the Holbeach shop was temporarily managed by a relief manager until a full time manager was appointed. That was a golden opportunity for me. Ken Exley, the relief manager, realised I had done no dispensing and I was way behind with the practical dispensing papers on the Boots course. He allowed me to stay late after the shop was closed and work my way through those practical exercises. The shop closed at 6pm, I used to work until about eight o'clock completing the dispensing papers, then I dropped the keys to Ken at his hotel before cycling back to Spalding. I also spent much more of my time during the day actually dispensing prescriptions.

Ken Exley, who was later appointed to the smaller Boots store in Grantham, became a very good friend. He recommended me to Colin Gunn, the head of the Leicester School of Pharmacy, and helped me obtain a place there to study. Ken had himself been a student at Leicester and was familiar with the department. He gave me a parting gift of a Chemistry book in which he had written a quote from the Rubaiyat of Omar Kyayyam -

'The Moving Finger writes; and, having writ,
Moves on: nor all thy Piety nor Wit
Shall lure it back to cancel half a line,'

This was very good advice for any student. It certainly warned me not to waste my time. Ken had been in the RAF during the war. The sentiments expressed in the Rubaiyat's verses had been adopted almost as a creed by the RAF lads at that difficult time.

Ken also sold me a small motorbike he had purchased to do his locum rounds but didn't much use. I became the proud owner of a James 125cc, two stroke motorcycle, which I intended using to get me to and from Leicester at weekends when I went on to study there. I passed my test on it withing three months and have been an occasional motorcyclist ever since, eventually working my way up to a Triumph 650cc twin cylinder bike.

My two year apprenticeship passed quickly. I became an expert in the agricultural side of the business, able to recommend products for Potato blight, Tomato wilt, weed sprays for Cereal crops and all the other products we sold to the farmers. Thanks to Ken Exley I was also reasonably proficient in practical dispensing.

Dispensing in the fifties was very different from today's dispensing. The majority of the prescriptions were for mixtures. We made indigestion mixtures such as Mist. (Latin for Mixture) Magnesium Trisilicate and Mist Magnesium Trisilicate and Belladonna; cough mixtures such as Mist. Tussi Nig and Mist Ammon Chlor and Morph; preparations for cystistis such as Mist. Potassium Citrate and Mist. Potassium Citrate and Hyoscyamus.

5

There were strong mixtures for treating diarrhoea, such as Mist. Creta Aromat cum Opio or Mist. Kaolin and Morph. Other presentation were prepared as gargles, lotions, emulsions and drops. Most of these formulae are obsolete at the present day; some are no longer available. Bottles of medicines were sealed with corks in those days before the screw tops were introduced. Every pharmacy had a cast iron cork press in the dispensary so that corks too large for the bottle could be compressed to size. You only see these implements in antique shops these day! Tablets were dispensed in ordinary screw topped bottles or small cardboard cartons before the bottles with childproof tops came into use.

Most ointments and skin creams were made on the premises. It was a regular weekly task for me to make 7lbs of Pasta. (Paste) Zinc Oxide and Ichthammol, which was much used for skin conditions. This ointment was hard work to make, which was probably why the task fell to the apprentice. The ointment slab had to be heated on a radiator before attempting to incorporate the Ichthammol into the very stiff Zinc Oxide base, especially on a cold winter morning. It took hours of work with a spatula to completely disperse the Ichthammol and produce an elegant preparation, and it made my arms ache.

Another one of my morning tasks was to prepare a winchester of Aqua Chlorof Duplex (Double strength Chloroform Water) and a winchester of Aqua Menth Pip.(Peppermint water). The winchester was a bottle containing four pints of liquid and commonly used to hold bulk liquid preparations. Chloroform Water and Peppermint Water were the vehicles for many of the common mixtures we made and dispensed. Chloroform is only slightly soluble in water so making the preparation entailed vigorous shaking of the winchester until all traces of the chloroform had gone into solution.

Peppermint Oil, which was used to make Aqua Menth Pip, is also reluctant to dissolve in water; another method had to be found to disperse it. I used to mix the oil with a little Talc to disperse it - (that is purified French Chalk) - The Talc then had to be filtered from the peppermint water before it could be used. We always had a winchester of both preparations in use and one of each as a spare supply.

The shop also still made some of its own brand products for sale. This was a legacy of the wartime when many items were scarce and even lipsticks were made in store. We produced two kinds of hand care preparations, which I made up in bulk. The cosmetic one was a pink gel made from Tragacanth, a gum used to thicken and suspend medicinal ingredients. I made a winchester of this hand gel with a little red Amaranth Solution added to give it a pink colour, and cologne added to perfume it.

Tragacanth makes a smooth gel if you know how to use it. It is first suspended in a little alcohol and rotated to thinly coat the sides of the glass winchester, water is then poured in quickly and the bottle shaken at once. Any hesitation produces a lumpy mess! We had a relief manager on one occasion who took the task from me and wasted a complete winchester of the lotion by not working quickly enough. His hand cream was too lumpy to be used.

The other hand cream we made was a more useful product used by local workmen in the winter. The carpenters and builders swore by this product, which had a more complicated formula based on Olive Oil, Lanolin and Lanette Wax. The preparation involved melting and mixing the oily ingedients over a hot water bath.

In my apprentice days, prescription labels were hand written with the occasional, ready printed, warnings attached to the containers. Such warnings as 'Shake the Bottle' or 'For external use only' were commonly used.

Boots supplied pads of the most common dispensing labels bearing instructions like 'One tablespoonful to be taken three times a day' or 'One to be taken twice a day', with the branch address printed on them. These ready printed labels saved time in a busy dispensary as all the dispenser needed to do was write the date and the name of the patient on the label before affixing it onto the product. Anything unusual had to be handwritten onto a blank label. The backs of the labels were coated with a water soluble glue and wetted on a sponge or roller before applying them to the containers, unlike the self adhesive ones in use today.

Prescriptions were ordered and made up using the Apothecary weights and measures system. The Apothecary or Troy ounce was divided into eight 60 grain drachms, twentyfour 20 grain scruples, and 480 grains. The liquid ounce was divided into 480 minims and eight 60 minim drachms. The usual dose volume for mixtures was One Tablespoonfull, which was equivalent to half a fluid ounce. The paediatric dose of One Teaspoonful was equivalent to one fluid drachm - this is equivalent to the 5ml dose volume we use today. These weights and measures had been used for generations and were well understood by the doctors and the pharmacists, but great changes were on the way.

When the prescriptions were completed they were wrapped very professionally in White Demi paper and sealed with red Sealing Wax. Bottles of mixtures were a difficult shape to wrap expertly and much practise was necessary to get an elegantly finished product to hand to the patient. The necessary folds in the wrap were accentuated by using the blade of a steel spatula. I learned the standard way of doing this task but a few years later was shown a more elaborate 'Wing Collar' wrap by an elderly dispenser who had been taught it years before. It belonged to a more elegant age. In today's busy dispensaries where most of the preparations are tablets or capsules and contained in

8

carboard boxes, the use of the ubiquitous dispensing bag is the most sensible way to present the prescriptions, but a nostalgic link with pharmacy's past has been lost.

When I studied at Leicester School of Pharmacy in the 1950s the profession was already preparing itself for the introduction of metric measures. The modern 5ml dose was on the horizon. On the pharmacy course we learned to use both systems and to interchange them.

Later when the metric system was officially adopted, pharmacists were forbidden by law to use the old apothecary system. (The British Parmacopoea changed to metric in 1963). Unfortunately, parliament decided that some older doctors might have a problem changing their habits so they were allowed to order in either system. The chemist had the task of translating their efforts! I recall many prescription written in a mixture of apothecary and metric measurements. Some prescriptions were written with ingredients in grains and drachms as well as milligrams and millilitres and the dose volume stated as half a ounce! Chemists soon became familiar with the equivalent weights and volumes in both systems and happily translated and accurately dispensed these hybrids

At about the time we changed weight and volume measurements the habit of writing the prescription in dog Latin began to change to plain English. In the fifties a code of abbreviations was used by doctors based on Latin, which had been the language of educated people throughout the Middle Ages. Instructions such as i t.d.s, - which was short for 'i ter in die sumendus' - (meaning one to be taken three times a day) were used on all prescriptions. Occasionally a private prescription from an older doctor would be presented with the formula and instructions written in full Latin. Those were an anachronism but a pleasure to see and dispense.

With the introduction of the National Health Service and the standardised prescription forms, English instructions slowly became the norm, as they are to this day. I wonder what the present day pharmacy graduate would make of those old prescriptions? If they could be read and understood, I suspect the preparation would be handed over to a Specials Manufacturing Unit and not prepared secundum artem (according to the art) in the dispensary, as we used to do. The profession has changed completely. The art of dispensing preparations has been lost as the vast majority of prescriptions are for ready-made dose forms such as capsules or tablets, which only require counting and labelling once they are checked for dosage, incompatability etc. The pharmacist is now becoming the expert on medicine use but I feel the pharmacy profession is still trying to understand its role in the modern health service as things are changing so rapidly. Successive governments have tampered with the National Health Service and often the changes have not been for the better.

The history of pharmacy has always been one of change. The old apothecaries used to diagnose their patients needs and charge them to make up the necessary medicines, while the doctors charged for the expertise of diagnosing the problem, often relying on Astrology as a diagnostic tool, and had the medicine made up by an assistant. Eventually the apothecaries concentrated on the dispensing and supply of medicines and became pharmacist, while the doctors stuck to diagnosis. Of course, surgeons started as Barber Surgeons who would do blood letting and few other surgical procedures.

The history of our health care system is fascinating and ever changing. Today Pharmacists are taking on extra tasks like blood pressure checks, influenza vaccinations, patient medicine reviews and advising doctors on what medicines to use. In hospitals the pharmacist has become a regular member of the medical team. In retail, some Pharmacists have become prescribing chemists, writing and issuing prescriptions to patients from a limited list of preparations. Plus ca change!

Chapter Two - The Apprenticeship

When I first started work at Boots store in Holbeach I struck up an immediate friendship with the shop porter, Ernest Scampion, known to all locally as Scamp. He had been a policeman in the area before he retired and knew practically everybody in the town and surrounding coutryside. He was a useful chap to know. As local bobby he had many contacts and often came to work bearing a brace of Pheasant, which some local farmer had given him. He was also a keen home brewer. Boots, like many chemists at that time, used to sell the materials for home brewing. We stocked demijohn jars, fermentation air locks, filter papers and funnels. Dried hops, malt and dried brewer's yeast were also sold as ingredients for beermaking. Kits containing all the necessary ingredients were quite popular but many of the home brewers prefered their own concoctions. Scamp produced a very nice imitation Sherry from raisons, corn, yeast and brown sugar. He gave me the recipe, which I tried and was quite pleased with the result. Of course, I only undertook brewing in the name of research, so I could advise the customers how to go about it.

Between us, Scamp and I dealt with all the deliveries; we wheeled in all the goods and unpacked them. We also delivered medicines and other items to the Fleet nursing home and to customers all over the village. The shop had a carrier bicycle for this purpose. I got to know the Holbeach area and its inhabitants very well during my two years there. There were many differences between a small village like Holbeach and a larger town like my home town of Spalding. I recall one evening leaving work and seeing a council vehicle slowly coming up the High Street, stopping occasionally at some of the premises. I stood talking to the porter before I cycled home to Spalding. As we talked I became aware of an unpleasant smell in the air.

"My! The airs a bit ripe this evening."

Scamp laughed out loud at my comment. "That would be the Bovril Boat coming up the High Street." He pointed to the council vehicle approaching us.

"Bovril Boat?"

"That's what the locals call it. It comes once a week to empty folk's toilets."

Further questioning elicited the fact that many of the older premises in Holbeach were still not on the mains sewer system and used outside toilets that needed emptying on a regular basis. I suppose many outlying fenland villages were like that in the 1950s.

Boots branch in Holbeach was situated in a three storey building immediately opposite to the church. The ground floor was the storage and sales area; the first floor was mainly staff quarters with the toilets, an office and a staff tea room; the top floor was little used. We also had a cellar beneath the sales area.

The cellar was reasonably cool so it was used to store some of the medicines that required such conditions. In the days before refrigerators were used in every pharmacy, we stored Insulin and Penicillin G injections down the cellar for a short time. The boss was also the recipient of many pheasants from his farming cronies. He hung these from the beams above the cellar steps to get high before he took them home to be cooked and eaten. On one occasion when I ran down the cellar to fetch an item for the dispensary, I remember feeling something cold drop down my shirt collar and wriggled down my back. When I checked, I found several live maggots, which had fallen off the Pheasant hanging above me! I am not a lover of Pheasant meat, maybe that is the reason why.

I spent a lot of my time on the shop counter serving customers. Being a small pharmacy we sold everything we stocked over the same short counter. Staff would serve customers with medicines, gardening items, toiletries and personal items all at the same time. The tills were rudimentary. There were no electronic cash registers in those days. Each till consisted of a wooden box with two drawers; one for change and one for bank notes. The receipts were hand written and in two parts; the top copy given to the customer and the carbon copy kept at the shop. It certainly sharpened your ability to add up when totalling many items under the scrutiny of the waiting customer. The bottom copies of the receipt books were sent off weekly to Boots head office where they were totalled and reconciled with the shop takings. Needless to say, if a mistake had been made it took so long for it to come to light there was no way to remember the circumstances.

Sometimes customers would request some strange sounding items. I recall on one occasion being asked for Barrack Sergeant's Drops. I checked with the dispensary and was told they were a controlled drug kept in the Dangerous Drug Cupboard. I was intrigued by this information and by the unusual name of the preparation. On researching it, I found Barrack Sergeant's Drops were taken for back ache. They consisted of Juniper Oil, Turpentine Oil and Tincture of Opium in Rectified Spirit. Twenty to thirty drops of the preparation were taken on sugar as a cure for Lumbago. I never forgot that particular preparation and wondered where it had got its exotic name.

Many of the preparation we stocked had names which would sound very odd to a modern pharmacist. We stocked Marshmallow Ointent and Grasshopper Ointment. Some of the customers would ask for even stranger items such as 'Three pennyworth of four haporths!' That was a cold remedy containing Sweet Spirits of Nitre among other ingredients. Sweet Spirits of Nitre was purchased as a diaphoretic - to sweat out a cold. Opodeldoc was another item frequently sold. That was the common name for Liniment of Soap, often refered to as Opidopi by many of the older customers. That was used to massage aching muscles, as was white oils and Grattons Embrocation, both these preparations were based on Turpentine Oil emulsion. Many of the customers would demand horse embrocation as they believed it must be a stronger preparation and more efficacious for their back aches.

In the back shop I was responsible for cleaning the shelves and the glass containers so I could become familiar with the names of the items stored there and their doses. On those shelves we stocked items such as Sanguine Dragonis - powdered Dragons Blood, which sounded prehistoric but was just a red colouring matter. We also stocked Venice Turpentine, a resin product from pine trees, which was used to make paints. As well as all the wet and dry drugs used in the dispensing of the medicines, country chemists in those days stocked many items, which were not of a medical nature.

We had one gentleman customer who would leave a small suitcase at the store to be filled with his listed preparations for making his own brand of furniture polish. His list included such items as beeswax, soft soap and turpentine oil, from which he manufactured a polish to sell to the local public houses for polishing their counter tops and their wooden drinks tables. I regularly got the job of weighing out and measuring his list of ingredients. I was surpised he could make a living doing that job.

All the wet and dry drugs had Latin names, which I had to familiarise myself with. Even common items such as White and Yellow Beeswax were labelled in Latin as Cera Alb. and Cera Flav. Latin was a language I had studied at school but that was little help in understanding the pharmaceutical version of it.

Another liquid preparation we kept in a wets cupboard in the stock room was Tincture of Cantharidine also know as Spanish Fly. That was yet another strange name. I found out that preparation was made from cantharis vesicatoria, a dried beetle. I never saw a prescription for the item but understand it was used as a counter irritant, but it was frowned upon as it caused blistering and was dangerous if absorbed through the skin. I have no idea why that tincture was stocked in the Holbeach store; maybe it was used in some veterinary preparation. After a time I became aware of Spanish Fly's other reputation as an aphrodisiac, but I never could understand why anyone would use such a dangerous substance for that purpose.

Some of the more unusual farming and gardening items requested by customers took me completely by surprise. I remember a farmer asking me for a gallon of Pig Oil. At that time I wasn't sure if pigs needed oiling and wondered if perhaps they had arthitic joints. I wondered if the preparation was actually made from pigs or whether it was just an unusual name for a product. I soon learned that Pig Oil was a grade of Light Liquid Paraffin, which was used to rub onto the pigs' skins to make them presentable for showing at an agricultural show. We sold it in gallon tins so there must have been many spruced up pigs in the Lincolnshire shows.

Another surprising gardening product that we stocked was flower dye. I believe this is still used today. White, Daisy type, flowers were cut and their stems placed in a solution of Faierie Flower dye. The colour soaked up the stems and dyed the white petals. The dyes were available in all of the primary colours. White Estereeds were commonly grown in the area and dyed in this way to make them more decorative.

As so much of he business at the Holbeach store was in the horticulture department, I was employed as a Farms and Gardens assistant and not trained properly as an apprentice pharmacist. My boss spent many hours in the Cheques Inn, next door to the shop, where he would meet his farming clients and increase the business.

The second world war had finished in 1945 but it threw a long shadow over the next few years. This was brought home to me when one afternoon I was searching through some old paperwork and stumbled across the Saccharin Register. Sugar was rationed during the second world war and was one of the last items to be taken off rationing as late as 1953. The chemist shop had managed to obtain regular supplies of saccharin tablets during the war years and had sold them in packets of 100 tablets to its regular customers. The demand for this sweetener was so great the manager had had to ration their supply and keep a register of named customers so the distribution was fair. This brought home to me how recent the war and rationing had been, and what a large range of things had been affected by the shortages. As a child born before the war started, I had lived through those hard times but regarded them as normal. Now the country was recovering very slowly from those lean years the deprivation became more obvious.

Chapter Three - Poisons!

During my apprenticeship I soon realised the pharmacist was in a privileged position with the ability to supply both medicines and poisons. I mention in another chapter many of the noxious substances we handled on a daily basis. The business was carried out under the Pharmacy and Poisons Act of 1933, which still defined the law as it applied to pharmacy in the early 1950s. The act had seventeen schedules defining the types of poisons and the systems applying to them. The most noxious substances were in the first schedule and were refered to as S1 poisons. The medical substances, which came under this law, were in Schedule Four and referred to as S4 substances. As chemists in a rural area, Boots at Holbeach carried many poisons, which were used in farming. I have mentioned some of them before but will elaborate on that list.

Cyanide was stocked as the Sodium salt. Cymag powder was the bulk of this trade but we did stock and sell small solid balls of Sodium Cyanide sealed in glass jars. This was used to destroy wasps nests. The cyanide ball was pushed into the nest and left to do its job. This difficult task was usually carried out after dark when the insects were not active. I was curious as an apprentice and unscrewed the lid of one of these jars; the cyanide had a distinctive, bitter almond, odour.

We also sold a poisonous alkaloid called Brucine. It sold in sachets called Molrat and was a similar chemical to Strychnine. We occasionally even sold Strychnine itself. These alkaloids were both used to kill moles. Under the regulations in force at the time, Strychnine could also be

18

sold to kill Seals, but I don't recall a call for it for that purpose at the Holbeach store. The method used for killing Moles was simple enough. The alkaloid was placed in a jar with several live earth worms. These were shaken together to coat the worms in the poison then they were put back into the soil in the hope the Moles would eat them and die.

I do recall one afternoon meeting the local Mole catcher at the shop. He used Mole traps, which were spring loaded devices sunk into the ground in one of the animal's regular subterranean passages. He used those rather than resorting to the more expensive and dangerous practice of using poison. I was intrigued at the idea of mole catching and had a few discussions with him about his job, which he told me was a family affair; his father and grandfather had been Mole catchers before him. His father, he assured me, used to sport a Moleskin waistcoat. I marvelled at how many skins it would take to make a whole waistcoat, as the Mole is such a small animal! Once or twice I had skinned and set up moles when I was practising my hobby of taxidermy. They were very small creatures. To make a waistcoat each soft fury skin would have to be preserved to leather then they would be sewn together to form a sheet of material. The front of the garment would have been made from this material. It must have taken many hours and much skill to skin and preserve that number of Moles let alone make them into a man's waistcoat.

As well as Mole traps and poisons many of the customers who were plagued by Moles in their lawns and gardens swore by a simpler deterrents. I was assured Moth Balls were the answer! They would buy the naphthalene balls and put a few down each of the moles underground tunnels. Presumably, the Moles didn't like the smell. I can't swear to the efficacy of this method of Mole control but it was quite popular in the 1950s.

Another poison we regularly stocked was Nicotine Sulphate spray, which was used to kill greenfly on plants. This was very poisonous, which begs the question why anyone would want to smoke tobacco and take such a substance into their lungs!

We also stocked Paris Green, which was used to kill slugs. Paris Green, was an arsenical; chemically it was Copper Acetoarsenite. This poison came as a free flowing, bright green, powder. We stocked this poison in a large drum and used to fill smaller containers from this bulk supply. To reduce the amount of handling the arsenical, the porter and I used to pour the Paris Green out of the large drum through a piece of rubber inner tube to funnel it into the smaller containers. The fine green powder flowed freely, almost like a liquid. Farmers would purchase this product, mix it with bran or cereal seeds and broadcast it on the fields to kill the slugs and snails.

The usual slug destroyer in those days contained Metaldehyde made into medium sized pellets. This chemical attracted slugs and snails but was fatal to them. I recall on one occasion we supplied a hundredweight sack of this slug destroyer to a farmer but he wasn't satisfied with it. When he broadcast the product over his crop of Tulips, the flower heads were bruised by the pellets making the crop unsaleable. My boss had the bright idea of crushing the pellets to a powder so we didn't lose the sale. The porter and I spent hours working in the open yard behind the shop. We spread the pellets onto sheets of brown paper and pounded them to a powder with a 28lb iron weight. We worked outside to avoid breathing in the fine dust that was produced but we still felt rather nauseous; this was one effect of breathing in Metaldehyde dust.

As Chemists in that area of the Lincolnshire fens, we also sold an organic Mercury product, which was used to sterilise Bulbs. Tulip and Daffodil bulbs were prone to damage caused by Eelworms and had to be treated after they were lifted from the ground in the autumn. Eelworms are a tiny nematode worm that eats and damages the bulb crops. They also attack potatoes. Soil carrying the infestation can only be used for resistant crops until the pest is completely eradicated.

When I worked on the land after leaving school I was involved in this bulb sterilising work. We used to immerse the bulbs, held in large wire cages, into a huge vat of the hot solution. It was heavy work. The operatives wore large rubber aprons and elbow length rubber gloves. Eventually, in spite of this treatment, much of the land around the Spalding area became infected with Eelworms and was no longer used to cultivate Tulips and Daffodils.

Schedule One poisonous substances could only be sold to the public under stricted conditions. The purchaser must be known to the pharmacist as a person to whom the poison may properly be sold, or the buyer must present a certificate signed by a householder known to the seller as a responsible person of good character. Failing these two alternatives, a certificate signed by a householder and endorsed by a police officer in charge of a police station would suffice. In a small community like Holbeach the pharmacist usually knew personally all the customers who had a need to purchase such poisonous substances. The pharmacist then filled in the Poisons Register and the customer signed the entry. The certificates had to be retained in the store. S4 substances could only be supplied to the general public against a prescription issued by a duly qualified medical practitioner, a registered dentist or a registered veterinary surgeon or practitioner.

The regulations were thorough, covering such topics as storage, labelling, containers, transporting, colouring and recording of the substances involved. The form of paperwork, such as prescriptions and signed orders, was regulated in great detail.

Chapter Four - Cyanide for Rodent Destruction.

One day early in my apprenticeship at Boots store in Holbeach my boss shouted for me as I was weighing out some cough candy in the back shop. "There's an urgent parcel coming on the bus from Wisbech. Go and pick it up."

I washed my hands and made to leave the shop.

"You'd better take the wheels. It's a heavy one."

I went and collected the sack barrow then wheeled it to the bus stop where the Wisbech bus was just arriving.

"Parcel for the chemists?" I asked the conductor.

"Under there." He pointed to a large wooden crate lodged on its end under the stairs, which led up to the top deck of the bus.

It was a heavy crate and I needed some help getting it from the bus platform and onto my wheels. Finally I pushed it back towards the shop, wending my way carefully between the pedestrians on the sidewalk. As I pushed the crate I couldn't help noticing a large label fixed to it with a Skull & Crossbones design on it. Beneath this warning logo was the word Poison. I was intrigued. This was a large consignment of poison and hardly the kind of product or the quantity a small chemist's shop would need. Back at the pharmacy my curiosity was soon satisfied.

"Take it round the back to the poison store and unscrew it." My boss ordered.

I undid the wooden lid and found eight tins of Cymag* inside the crate.

I knew what Cymag was because I had read the warning poster on the front of the poison store. It was a powder containing Sodium Cyanide and it must be kept dry because it generated deadly hydrogen cyanide gas if it came into contact with moisture. The sign on the outside of the poison store was a warning to the fire brigade that they must take precautions if they used water to quench a fire in that area!

I unpacked the eight large tins of poison and placed them on the shelves beside the other deadly substances we stored there. There were small jars of Sodium Cyanide for destroying wasp nests, packets of strychnine for killing moles and a large drum of Paris Green; an arsenical compound, which was mixed with grain and broadcast on the tulip fields to kill the slugs. Country chemist shops sold these items to the farmers on a regular basis in the 1950's.

"That's an awful lot of Cymag." I said.

"Aye. The rodent disposal men are collecting it today. It's for the sea walls. The regular carrier doesn't come until next week. That's why we had to get an emergency supply sent over quickly on the bus."

We locked the poison store and I washed my hands but I couldn't contain my curiosity. "What do they do with all that poison on the sea walls?".

"They use it to kill rats and rabbits that burrow into the earth banks. If they went unchecked the earth banks would collapse and the sea would flood the fens again."

This explanation made perfect sense to me. Holbeach was a fen village protected from the encroachment of the North Sea by wide and high earth banks. If these sea walls were not kept in good order that whole area of the Lincolnshire fens would be flooded and returned to the sea. People's homes, farmers' crops and livestock would all be lost. There could even be loss of life.

Later that afternoon two men called at the pharmacy. They were father and son dressed in scruffy

24

outdoor clothes, typical of labourers wo king on the land.
I helped them load the tins of Cymag into their open
backed truck while the chemist filled in the poison register
and checked their permit from the Ministry of Agriculture.

"This amount should last you ages." I said

"No lad. We have no end of rats in the banks. We'll
be back next week for another load."

I watched them as they drove off along the fen road.
They did indeed call the next week for another half
hundredweight of the cyanide poison. Curiosity got the
better of me. "How do you get the rabbits to take this?" I
think I naively had visions of them dipping carrots in the
poison and putting them down the burrows.

The older man laughed out loud. "We don't dose
them, lad. We gas them down their holes."

"Oh!" I felt stupid having asked the question. "Any
chance I could see you doing it? On my half day?"

"Of course. Come over to the sea bank and we'll
show you how we work. You being into chemistry, you'll
be interested."

I cycled out to the fen on the Thursday afternoon
and found the pair of them working along the sea bank.
They seemed only too pleased to explain their work to me.

"We put the cyanide down the hole with this." The
son held up a long cane with an ordinary tablespoon tied
onto the end of it with string. He dipped the spoon into an
open tin of Cymag and filled the bowl with the powder.
"That goes down the hole."

I watched, fascinated but concerned. There was a
breeze blowing across the fen and some of the white
cyanide powder blew into the air from the container and the
spoon. I moved away to avoid the poison.

"That's right, keep upwind of it, lad." The father said.
"It's nasty stuff."

25

Nasty stuff! I remember thinking there was probably enough cyanide in those tins to kill the entire population of Holbeach! I watched as the son put the spoon down the rat hole then turned it over to deposit the contents deep underground. When he had withdrawn the spoon he sealed the hole with a sod of earth and moved on to the next one.

"The damp in the soil reacts with the powder and gives off a poisonous gas. That kills anything down the hole," he explained.

I walked along the sea bank searching for rat and rabbit holes as I went. I found there were indeed hundreds of them on that small stretch of coastline.

Next day at the shop I was approached by the firm's farming representative with an unusual request. I had started practising a bit of taxidermy in those days as a hobby, having helped at the local museum while I was at school, and learned something of the art.

"Any chance you could stuff a few rats for me?" Norman asked.

"Yes…Why?"

He laughed. "I could use them on a display at the agricultural stand. It will help me sell more rat poison."

Norman covered a large area of the fenland selling agro-chemicals to the farmers. He regularly stood a stall on Wisbech market to do this.

"I'll have to get some dead rats first." I told him, but I already had an idea who to ask.

Next week when the rodent men came to collect the Cymag I had a word with them. "I could do with a couple of dead rats to stuff. I'd like some large, well coated specimens"

They thought this very odd, until I explained what I wanted them for. "Ok lad. We'll see what we can do. I suppose you'd like nice big uns?"

I nodded, then watched them drive off along the fen

road with the Cymag in the back of their truck.

I saw nothing of the rodent operatives for several weeks after that. I'm sure they came to the shop but I was always elsewhere at the time. Then, one afternoon as I was dusting the drug bottles in the back shop, I heard a loud scream. I was called urgently into the sales area by my irate boss.

"Get that sack out of the shop," he bellowed.

I hurried into the shop, picked up a heavy sack and carried it into the yard. The dispenser, a rather refined young lady, followed me outside and waved her fist at me.

"They left that by the dispensary and I opened it to check what it was! Then they told me it was for you."

By this time I had opened the sack to reveal it was full of large dead rats. I couldn't help but smile. I would have given a week's wages to see the dispenser's face when she opened that sack. It served her right for being so nosey. Of course, there were far too many dead rats for my purpose so I picked out the largest two and threw the remainder in the dustbin.

A few weeks later, when I'd had time to set up the specimens and they had dried, I presented Norman with his two sales aids.

"Lovely. Just what I wanted." He admired the rats set up on their wooden bases. One, I had set standing normally and the other I had posed sitting up with a knife and fork in its paws and a bib around its neck. I had used that rather macabre pose for the specimen so the farmers would really get the message of how much of their profits were eaten by rats. As a reward for me, Norman told the boss he needed a hand on his stall that afternoon so I went with him to the cattle market and helped him set out his display and serve the farmers. It was a welcome change from the routine of the shop.

The rats were a success. Several people took a second

27

look when they spotted them on our stall, perched on top of tins of rat poison. A few passersby stood and stared for several minutes, probably waiting for them to move! Norman was thrilled with my work as they provided a talking point and gave him the opportunity to discus the merits of our rat poison. When the market ended I put the rats in a shallow box and carried them back to Norman's car. It was very crowded, but the public parted and let me through as soon as they spotted what I was carrying.

A few days later, back at the shop, I mounted a window display of agro-chemicals with the rats and rat poison in a prominent place. I placed a plate of grain in front of the specimen wielding the knife and fork, to reinforce the message. It stopped many of the locals when they happened to glance into that window.

I got to know the rodent men quite well during my two year apprenticeship. They were always kept busy keeping the sea walls free of rats and rabbits. A few years later, after I had qualified as a pharmacist, I worked at Holbeach for a short time. I asked after the rodent men and was sorry to hear the father had died and his son was a sick man. I remember wondering if their constant use of Cyanide had affected their health adversely. On reflection, it is obvious Health and Safety considerations were not a priority in my apprentice days.

* *The use of Cymag was banned in 2004.*

Chapter Five - Time at College

My college years at Leicester were busy. The pharmacy course was bursting at the seams with content. The main subjects studied were Dispensing, Phamacognosy (the study of medicinal plants), Pharmaceutical Chemistry, Human Physiology, Forensic Pharmacy (the study of the pharmacy law), Pharmaceutics (the manufacturing of products), Pharmacology (the study of drug action) and Microbiology. Most of these subjects were studied in theory in lectures and at a practical level in the laboratories.

Lincolnshire County paid my fees and granted me £120 a year towards my other costs. That princely sum just about covered the cost of my books so I had to work every holiday to afford my digs, to eat and to pay all my other expenses like running my motorbike and buying clothes. I put myself through college with a little help from Lincolnshire County.

When I went away to college I still had 3 months of my apprenticeship to complete so the first three months of my holidays were spent at Boots Holbeach completing that period of training. After that three month period was over, I worked for Boots as a relief dispenser for some of the holiday times and worked on the land for the remainder of it. I was fortunate in always finding work and I managed to pay my own way through the pharmacy course. I even bought a larger motorbike as the constant journeying between Leicester and Spalding, a round trip of about 100 miles every weekend, eventually proved too much for the small 125cc James I had bought from Ken Exley.

I part exchanged that two stroke bike and bought a

larger, four stroke, BSA, motorbike, which did the trip in far less time. I finished my pharmacy course with no debts, but no savings either.

The reasons I went home to Spalding each weekend were many. It meant I paid less for my digs in Leicester, it also meant I could get my washing done free of charge at the weekends and I could see my mother and my girlfriend. Those regular breaks helped to pass the three years I was studying. Because of the amount of studying on the pharmacy course we worked late one evening per week in the laboratories and we had a lecture on Saturday morning. This Saturday lecture delayed my trip home each weekend so I had a word with the head of department, Mr Colin Gunn.

Mr Gunn lectured us on Pharmaceutics on the Saturday mornings. I soon realised he was reading the lecture verbatim from his own textbook - Tutorial Pharmacy by Cooper and Gunn. He had obviously used that text for some years because he had pasted the pages onto foolscap sheets of paper and written his jokes and comments on the margins! I bought his book and told him I would read the relevant pages at home over the weekend as I wouldn't be able to make the lectures. Mr Gunn was quite alright with this arrangement and I made sure I kept to my side of the bargain as I would have exams to pass in the subject. Once that arrangement was in place, I drove home each Friday evening and back to Leicester on the following Sunday night, whatever the weather, making the break worthwhile.

The A47, the main road I took from Leicester, is a road with many steep hills. I do remember one hard winter driving up Wardley Hill near Uppingham on my way home to Spalding. Before that hill was improved in 1987 it was long, steep and winding.

That winter there had been heavy snow in the area. The road had been cleared to leave a single vehicle track with occasional passing places cleared to one side of it. The snow was piled higher than my head ; it was like riding between high white walls with no sight of the surrounding countryside. I rode my motorbike up that hill with a leg held out at each side to prevent the bike skidding. It was often a hair raising journey home but I didn't miss one weekend in the whole three years, whatever the weather; rain, hail or snow.

One dark night going back to Leicester, the bike skidded on wet leaves. I landed in the middle of the road with the BSA on top of me. It was a heavy bike but I soon moved it off me in case a lorry came along in the dark. Desperation can give you strength!

The only serious accident I had while motorcycling was in Spalding. I was hit by a car, which came out of a side road without stopping. That accident only bruised me and gave me gravel rash on my face but it bent the front forks of the bike making it unusable. That weekend I had to catch a bus back to Leicester. The following weekend with my motorbike repaired but still in Spalding, I pedalled my pushbike the 50 miles home so I could collect it.

My time at Leicester passed quickly and enjoyably. The group of students I joined were a nice bunch of men and women. Leicester attracted many Welsh students at the time, probably because the city's director of education, a Mr Thomas, was himself Welsh. On social occasions, like bus journeys to and from Rugby matches, the Welsh contingent always gave voice to their songs. They lived up to their reputation as a nation of choirs! Many's the time we were serenaded by Sospan Fach and other Welsh language songs. Some of the ditties I swear were made up on the spot. I do recall one which went something like :-

"I have a brother Trevor and they say he's very clever.
And to gain more knowledge he did go to Leicester College.
Did you ever saw.
Did you ever saw
Did you ever saw such a funny thing before."

There were inumerable verses to this song, the rest of which I have forgotten, but it did pass the time on a boring bus journey.

We worked hard and occasionally broke the monotony with a trip organised by the pharmacy department. The one which stands out for me was a trip to the Coventry Theatre to see The Goons. Peter Sellars, Spike Milligan and Harry Secombe made the theatre rock with laughter. They were popular in the 50's and became radio legends. My personal favourite was Spike. His humour was in tune with my student mind.

Exams, of course, came around far too often. After a year the first external examination was held in Nottingham; Leicester College was not an exam centre for pharmacy in those days. The final exam, taken two years later, was held at Manchester University.

I rode up to Manchester on my motorbike and stayed at the YMCA for the three week period of the exams. Little did I realise the railway station was situated immediately behind the YMCA and the whole night would be interrupted by the noise from the taxi ranks next to the building. Someone kept blowing a whistle to summon the taxis so I got little sleep the first night.

Manchester University laboratories caused a few practical problems for we Leicester students. Much of the glassware and laboratory equipment was different from what we had grown used to at Leicester. It did add to the stress of the final examinations. One or two of my fellow students, people I regarded as sure of passing the exams, failed them and had to take refers at a later date.

I received my succesful results on August 1st 1958 an l paid my registration fee of £1 to the Pharmaceutical Society for the remainder of that year. I was then registered as a Pharmaceutical Chemist and a Member of the Pharmaceutical Society, able to legally be in charge of a pharmacy.

My fiancee and I had known each other since our school days and had been engaged for three years. We had planned to get married if I was successful. We married on August 16th. knowing I was due for National Service and planning to bank the marriage allowance to increase our savings.

Chapter Six - Locum Work & Relief Management

After I passed my examination and registered with the Pharmaceutical Society, I knew I was due to be called up for National Service. The government had allowed students to postpone their National Service until after they had finished their education, so I started my Service at the age of 21 instead of the normal 18 years of age. My fiancee and I had been engaged for nearly three years and decided to get married before I went into the RAMC. We married at Spalding Parish Church on the 16th of August 1958.

I spent the three months between the August and the November, when I was due in the army, doing relief management for Boots in the Eastern area, based at my home in Spalding. It was an interesting time for me. I managed branches in Skegness and Wisbech and spent a lot of time at the Spalding store where the manager, Derek Offer, was very kind and allowed me to bring my management knowledge up to scratch. On November the 5th I reported to Crookham Barracks in Hampshire for my basic training in the RAMC.

My time in the RAMC only lasted 6 months. I developed a shoulder problem, which made it too painful to lift my arms, even to salute a superior officer! At the time they put it down to repetitive strain caused by such tasks as carrying bodies on stretchers over high walls and similar exercises we were expected to do in training. I was taken off the basic training a week before I would have completed it and was put onto pharmacy duties in the camp medical centre. If I had completed the basic training then been discharged from the army, I may have been due a pension and that they wanted to avoid.   No proper diagnosis was made at the time but a few years later, when it was investigated properly, I was diagnosed with osteoarthrits in my spine and I knew the true cause.   As the specialist succinctly put it. "You've chosen the wrong parents. Your spine xrays look like a navvy in his forties!"   It was a hereditary problem, which made it very painful to sit for any length of time as my worn vertebrae trapped nerves such as my sciatic nerve. I was fortunate that my chosen profession involved standing up all the time.

After my time in the RAMC I returned to Spalding to find Boots had reorganised their Territories and   the Spalding branch had been transfered from the Nottingham area to the Leicester area; from T1 to T2. I was offered the choice of areas and decided to join T2 based in Leicester as I had lived in that city for three years while I studied pharmacy and I was very familiar with the area.

When I rejoined Boots I was based at their Gallowtree Gate store in Leicester for six months to catch up on my dispensing knowledge; it is surprising the changes that had happened while I was away in the army.

The store had late opening hours until nine at night and had a very busy dispensary. I was part of one of the teams that manned the late night service.   There were usually four members in a team, a pharmacist, a dispenser and two counter staff to serve the customers and to receive and give out the prescriptions on the chemist counter. The dispensary at the Gallowtree Gate store in those days was on the first floor and removed from the public view. It was situated immediately above the chemist counter. We had a small service lift connecting to the counter area. This carried the prescription forms up to the dispensary and the completed prescriptions   down to the   staff who were manning the counter.

This system meant the dispensing staff were relatively immune from the hurly burly of the store but if there was a dispensing query from a customer, one of us had to go downstairs to answer it.

When I completed my pharmacy qualification, I realised my handwriting was atrocious thanks to speed writing when taking the massive volume of notes necessary on the pharmacy course. In those days prescription labels were hand written and it was essential the patients could read the instructions on them. I was so ashamed of my writing I decided to teach myself Italic writing to rectify the situation. I purchased a book that taught the system and set about learning it. It took me about three weeks to rid myself of my former bad habits and write clear and elegant Italic script. I bought myself a Swan Caligraphic pen and a bottle of black ink and never looked back. I still write Italic script to this day and can't even remember the way I was taught to form my letters at school. I would recommend the idea to anyone whose writing is in need of improvement.

In the dispensary at the Gallowtree Gate store we did a fair number of private prescriptions as well as numerous National Health Service ones. Private prescriptions were entered in a large, leather bound ledger. One day I did so many private prescriptions I almost filled a double page of that book. My Italic writing looked so good the other dispensing staff would not write on the remaining part of the second page not wanting comparison with my writing, so the space was left blank.

Once my dispensing was up to speed, I undertook relief management based in Leicester where Boots had seven branches. I also covered the rest of the territory replacing managers who were away on holiday or off ill.

It was on one of these duties I found the store dustbin full of Shop Rounds. The traditional glass containers used for storing medical chemicals that all chemists used to display on their dispensary shelves, were referred to as Shop Rounds. The jars for solids and the bottles for liquid preparations were made in clear glass, or coloured glass such as green or blue if they were to contain substances prone to degrade in daylight. There were also green or brown glass bottles with ribbed sides, which distinguished them as containers for poisonous ingredients, being identifiable by touch as well as appearance. Each of those containers had a glass label with a white background and black lettering declaring the name of the contents, and glass stoppers. Many of the labels were outlined in gold leaf, making them very decorative. Eventually chemist did not use such containers, prefering to use the bottles the chemicals are supplied in and recycling the empty bottles when they are replaced with a new one. This ensures new stock was not inadvertantly filled over old stock, which could lead to the older chemical degrading with age.

I searched through the rubbish bin behind the store and removed several of the old bottles and jars that had been thrown out. I still travelled by motorcycle in those days and saved as many of the obsolete Shop Rounds as I could get into my saddie bags. Had I left them they would have been taken by the refuse collectors and thrown on the waste tip the very next day when the rubbish bins were emptied. Those jars and bottles I still posses. The cover of this book is based on a photograph I took of some of them. Even then, as a newly qualified pharmacist, I had an eye for items that would become antiques and valuable. Beautifully made jars labelled with exotic Latin names like, Syrup Marrub, Nux Areca, Lin Saponis Meth, or even Perfumes sold in bulk like Essence of New Mown Hay were evocative of a bygone age. One of the dispensers I met on my locum travels remembered girls calling at the pharmacy on a Saturday afternoon to purchase a small bottle of that perfume to apply before they went out on the Saturday night. Perfumes are not sold loose like that today.

Essence of New Mown Hay does sounds very exotic. It contained Oils of Bergamot and Rose Geranium along with Tinctures of Benzoin, Essence of Musk and Alcohol. The base was Tincture of Tonka Bean, which contains Coumarin. It would not have had a light floral perfume, but more a heavy, musky odour.

After six months based in Leicester I was transfered to Boots Rugby store where the manager was absent for some months recovering from a serious operation. This was a large shop with a recorded music department, a book department and a jewellery department as well as the usual photographic, chemist, farming and toiletries sections. I enjoyed the challenge and the pace of the business. My wife and I spent about eighteen months in Rugby then returned to live in Leicester where I was based at the large store in Gallowtree Gate once again. Even though that was a city centre store it did a fair amount of farming business in those days. Whenever I was working in the store and not needed for chemist duties I would go onto the farming department, where the supervisor, Betty Berry, could always do with some knowledgeable help.

Relief management was an interesting job. I worked in so many different environments, in village shops and city stores. The experience was invaluable and on the whole enjoyable but occasionally tragedy marred the experience.

I was working at one store when a policeman arrived with an empty tablet bottle. He was very officious.

"Do you recognise this?" The constable asked the young lady dispenser.

She coloured up red and nodded that she did. I took the bottle from the officer and read the label. The bottle had contained 60 Sodium Amytal sleeping capsules.

"What's the problem?" I asked.

"We just wanted confirmation." The policeman explained. "Your patient has killed himself by taking the whole lot in one go. He put the capsules in a piece of apple pie and ate them all."

It was obviously no fault of the dispenser but she was so shaken with the interview and the circumstances she burst into tears. I sent her home for the day to recover.

On another occasion the police came to a store I was managing and produced an empty bottle of Lysol disinfectant. Lysol contained Cresol in those days and was extremely caustic. The bottle bore the store address label so there was no mistaking its source. On that occasion it transpired a gentleman had drank the contents of the bottle and had killed himself. His body was found sprawled on his front lawn. On both occasions the police were only following procedures to ascertain everything about the deaths but it was upsetting for the staff involved. Thankfully those problems were very rare.

My relief management days continued for a few more years. I was interviewed for several Deputy Management positions in large store such as Northampton, Blackpool and Birmingham - the largest Boots in the country at that time. I was unsuccessful and was finally offered the management of the small branch in Uppingham. At first I was disappointed at the offer as I had ambitions to work in larger stores, but common sense prevailed; especially as the move took my wife and I nearer to our home town of Spalding where both of our mothers still lived. Both mothers were getting older and we were concerned to be able to get over to see them and back to our home in one day. Spalding was about 35 miles from Uppingham and adequately filled that criteria. Once I had settled into village life in Rutland I never regretted the choice.

As sole pharmacist in Uppingham, I soon became a

valued member of the community. I ran for office on the local parish council, was elected and served as a councillor for several years. My wife and I had been members of the Bowmen of Glen archery club when we lived in Leicester. We even shot at the Game Fair when it was held at Burleigh House near Stamford. That event saw us appear on the cover of the Shooting Times; not for our archery prowess but because we both shot bows left handed and made an unusual photograph. Thanks to the generosity of Uppingham School we formed a small archery club, which used part of their Middle Field as our butts.

The Uppingham Boots store is in a central location on the High Street. At that time it was the only pharmacy in the village and I was the only pharmacist, which meant I was on duty every day of the year apart from when I was on holiday. The shop opened for business at 9am and closed at 7pm after the evening dispensing duty. I had a half day off on Thursday but had to go back to work from 6pm to 7pm to do the dispensing duty. I was on duty every Sunday and Bank Holiday, including Christmas Day, usually from 12 noon to 1pm to offer a dispensing and medicinal service. As well as the regular hours, I was on call, day or night, for the supply of urgent prescription items. There was even one Bank holiday when I did the hour at Uppingham then went and did the hour at Oakham to help out Tom Atkins, the manager there, who was involved in the Oakham Flower Show. On that occasion I could boast I had done the Rota Duty for the entire county of Rutland. Not many pharmacist can say they have covered a whole county on their own!

When I took over the Uppingham shop I volunteered to help some of the local groups by acting as a booking office for some of their events. We sold tickets for the local amateur dramatic productions and even for the Farmers' Ball, which was held annually in the hall of the

Uppingham School This event was organised by local farmers who also arranged and held the Uppingham Fat Stock Show in the town's market place. My wife and I used to attend the Ball, being keen amateur dancers. It was a shock to see many of my farmer customers out of their rugged outdoor clothes and sporting dress suits and bow ties!

Uppingham Fat Stock show is unique. It is the only event of its kind still held in a town market place in temporary pens. The recent show in November 2014 was the 109th such show to be held there. The event has had a continuous run, with the exception of the war years and two years when Foot and Mouth regulation prevented it. It usually takes place on a Wednesday morning in November when the local farms show their best pigs, sheep and cattle. Stock is brought into the pens from about 7am, judging begins at 10am with prizes awarded by about 11.30am. There is a lot of friendly rivalry among the exhibitors and the prizes are valued as proof of farm stock well raised.

Nelsons, the local butcher's shop, which was only a few doors away from Boots' store, used to buy some of the prize beasts that were sold for slaughter, and displayed their awards in their front window. On many occasions that shop window was adorned with numerous coloured rosettes and the silver cup won by the prize exhibit. The Fat Stock show is one of the main events in the Uppingham town calendar and an event well worth a visit. It is a unique example of the country way of life in rural Rutland that still continues to this day.

I had only been at the Uppingham store a short time when the shop was refitted. Out went the old Mahogany fittings to be replaced by modern melamine units. We had a new, more open, shop front and all new fixtures.

In the old shop above each window display we had a large hanging glass globe filled with coloured water. This

41

type of display was typical of old chemist's shop up and down the country. The glass globes were decorative but they were a problem to empty and refill when the coloured water faded or became turgid. When the shop fitters removed these antique display pieces they were transported immediately to Boots head office where they had quite a collection of bygones.

Refitting and modernising was a trend happening all over the country as pharmacies were updated. The mahogany cupboard doors with their glass fronts were thrown out but I couldn't tolerate such waste so I took them home and built myself a small greenhouse in the back garden of my bungalow. It was definitely a cut above the average greenhouse! The old mahogany fittings had served the shop for many years. I doubt the modern melamine ones would last as long.

I have included two photographs in this book of the Uppingham shop. The earlier one looks to be about 1900 in date with a nod towards Art Nouveau decoration. There was a glass window immediately above the front door which still bore the legend 'Late of Savoury and Moore Chemist to the Queen' This refered to Cornelius Bayley, the chemist who sold the business to Boots. Mr Bayley worked in the London pharmacy and came to Uppingham reputedly to enjoy the coutryside and the Fox Hunting.

The later photograph shows the store after the refit and much as it appears to this day.

Dispensing at the Uppingham pharmacy was similar to what I had experience as an apprentice in Holbeach. Mixtures were still made up as needed but more ready-prepared dose forms such as tablets and capsules were being prescribed. The doctors' practice in Uppingham was a dispensing doctor practice, which was, and still is, common in country areas. The surgery was responsible for dispensing prescriptions for patients who lived outside a one mile limit from the village. Those patients living within the village area were served by the pharmacy. The doctors' dispensing was under the supervison of the doctors

One unfortunate product sticks in my memory from the early 1960s. Thalidomide was introduced in about 1957 in Germany and was even sold over the counter there. It soon became popular over here in Britain. It was introduced as a sedative tablet and was recommended for treating nausea during pregnancy, with devastating results. Thankfully I do not recall many prescription being issued in Uppingham for Thalidomide but it was commonly used in some other areas of the country and caused many deformities in babies.

Much of the prescription business was for antibiotics. Penicillin started the trend in 1945 when it had become available for general use. The Tetracyclines were introduced in 1955 and were a popular bacteriostatic. Penicillin V came into use in 1956. Many of these new products were introduced during my years studying to become a pharmacist and were soon in constant use.

Ampicillin was introduced in 1961 about the time I took over the pharmacy in Uppingham and Amoxycillin came into use in 1972 while I was still at that branch of Boots. The Sulphonamide antibacterial drugs had been in use some time before, so we had a constantly growing armoury against bacterial infections. These products along with the hundreds of other antibiotics introduced, revolutionised the treatment of bacterial infections but today we see an ever increasing problem caused by their overuse. Unfortunately, more bacteria have developed immunity to these preparations and few new antibiotics are being researched and made. We have seen the golden age of the successful treament of bacterial infections but now it could be ending. Overuse of the antibiotics we have, has curtailed their usefulness. The use of antibiotics in animal feeds has also come under fire. The crossover of resistant bacteria from farm animal stock is blamed for some of the problems now found in humans. We are entering a period of uncertainty in the treatment of bacterial infections. Hospital superbugs now cause concern for patients undergoing treatment in those institutions. If the antibiotics no longer work, we will see many more deaths from bacterial infections and medicine will be pushed back to earlier and more difficult times.

Chapter Seven - Mustard Gas!

When I first took over the management of Boots in Uppingham in the early 1960's, I made a thorough inventory of the store. In the back shop we had a lot of old stock and obsolete paperwork including labels dating back to the time before Boots took the store over. I found scores of old chemist labels from the days when chemist nostrums were prepared and labelled on the premises. These were very decorative and would be a collector's item on today's antique market. I worked my way along the shelves of wets and dries finding bottles with Latin names on their labels such as Tr. Asoefetida, and bags of dry drugs like Boracic flake and Red Ochre. These items were seldom found in city pharmacies but were part of the stock in trade of a country chemist.

Asoefetida was a foul smelling substance consisting of a resin from the roots of certain Umbelliferous plants found in Iran and Turkey. It had an odour, and probably a taste, like rotten onions! You may wonder why a country chemist would stock such a substance but its very foulness provides the answer. Asoefetida was made into an ointment with soft paraffin and a red colouring. This preparation was smeared onto chickens that were being feather pecked by the other birds. I would think one taste of Asoefetida and the offending bird wouldn't try again! I have also heard that this substance could be made into a nail varnish and put onto people's fingernails to stop them biting them, but I 've never had experience of that useage.

Boracic flake was used on ballroom floors. Spread a little of the flake onto a wooden floor and it becomes slippery enough to ensure the dancers glide around to the music; spread too much and they would probably slip over!

Red Ochre was used as red raddle to trace which ewes had been served by the ram. The red dye was rubbed onto the ram's stomach. He left a telltale mark on any ewe he mounted. This gave the shepherd an idea which ewes were pregnant and a clue to when they would lamb.

When I was searching one particular cupboard in the back shop I came across a surprising relic of the second world war. I found a small wooden box with no label on it. I took it out of the cupboard and over to the window to see it better. I was intrigued to see a crusty deposit around the lid. Curious at this find and finding no further clue to its contents, I prised the lid open and found inside the outer wooden box a metal cylider with even more dark brown efflorescence forming around the neck. Whatever chemical was in that container, it was unstable and breaking down. I unpacked the box carefully and discovered a leaflet describing the contents. Imagine my surprise and horror to discover it was a cylinder of Mustard Gas!

The enclosed leaflet headed 'War Gas Samples', gave all the precautions and instructions for handling that very dangerous substance. It listed the protective clothing to be worn and the routine for dealing with dangerous spillages; it even recommending concentrated Nitric Acid to clean any surfaces contaminated by the contents! The leaflet also mentioned a sample of Lewisite, which was a particularly nasty chemical weapon containing organoarsenic and caused severe blistering, but thankfully that cylinder was missing.

Concerned at my find, I contacted the previous branch manager, who had just retired, and asked him what he knew about the box.

"Oh! is that still there? It's been there since the war." He further explained.   "I was not called up to serve in the army in the war; being a chemist I was in a reserved occupation, however, I was drafted into the Home Guard as a Scientific Officer."

"I can understand that, but why did you have Mustard Gas on the premises?" I was amazed at the find and even more surprised it was still in the cupboard some 17 or so years after the war had ended.

"We used to practise taking some of the Mustard Gas out of the container and putting on our gas masks in preparation for a gas attack. It was so we had experience of it. Everyone thought such a gas attack was imminent in the early years of the war and we needed to be prepared."

I was astounded. It seems the Home Guard practised their gas warfare drill by risking gasing themselves! I could not believe my ears. "That does seem a dangerous game."

He laughed. "That's nothing. As the designated bomb disposal expert for the village I had a barrel of sand on the pavement outside the shop front. If an incendary bomb fell nearby I was supposed to pick it up and put it the sand barrel!"

I had not realised how amateurish the preparations had been on the home front in the early years of the last war. No doubt experience soon taught them some hard lessons.

The crust around the Mustard Gas cylinder indicated it was unstable and it could prove dangerous, so I decided I must contact the local police to get it removed and destroyed. As the new manager of the store, the safety of the staff and myself was uppermost in my mind. Uppingham police had no idea what to do with the cylinder and passed the query on to a local army unit, which seemed eminently sensible. A few days later this information bore fruit. An armoured vehicle drew up outside the shop front with several uniformed soldiers on board. They closed the High Street with barriers then came into the shop.

47

The sergeant in charge came into the pharmacy and explained. "We've come to remove the Mustard Gas, Sir."

I was taken aback at all these precautions. After all, that cylinder had sat in a wooden cupboard in the back shop for years with no problems. The cupboard had been in constant use storing farms and gardens stock and was visited by every member of my staff, almost on a daily basis. I took the sergeant through to the back shop and showed him where the cylcinder was stored.

"Stand back, Sir. Leave it to us. We will dispose of the risk."

One of the other soldiers donned a complete protective suit. He was covered from head to foot in what appeared to be a stout canvas oufit. To complete the ensemble he donned a helmet, which completely encased his head, and had a transparent visor at the front.

I watched fascinated as the man used a long pair of metal tongs to pick up the box containing the gas cylinder. Holding the Mustard Gas at arm's length he gently took it out to the waiting vehicle, walking slowly and carefully like someone carrying an unexploded bomb. Once outside, he deposited the gas container into a large metal box attached to the front of the vehicle then immediately locked it. He treated the sample with such respect it may as well have been an unstable explosive.

By this time the High Street was filling with curious people standing at the barriers, wondering what was going on at their local pharmacy. Waiting cars were backed up the steet as far as the eye could see. My staff were standing at the front windows peering out at the army unit and waving to people they recognised in the crowd.

The sergeant thanked me for reporting the find and gave me a signed receipt for it, which I still have.

It read -

'Received. 1 Box containing Sample of Mustard Gas.' and it was signed *' R. Marrit Sgt   (Sgt R. Marrit   Northco. Ammo. Inspectorate York).*

I still have the leaflet, which was in the box and I have kept that along with the signed receipt Both are illustrated in this book.

It seemed a long way to come all the way from York to Uppingham for that small cylinder but I suppose it was an unusual incident occuring so long after the hostilities of the Second World War had ended.

The sergeant stood to attention, clicked his heels and smartly saluted me. "We will see it gets destroyed safely, Sir. These things are very dangerous."

I chuckled at this show of respect then I stood in the shop doorway and watched the soldiers dismantle their barriers.

The armoured vehicle vanished slowly up the High Street and the curious crowd dispersed. The whole affair had given Uppingham something unusual to talk about on a quite afternoon. After it had calmed down, one or two regular customers came into the shop to find out exactly what had occurred. I told them it was some training stuff left over from the war. I did not mention the words Mustard Gas not wishing to cause a panic in the High Street or see lurid headlines in the local newspaper.

Chapter Eight - A Haunting?

One November morning in the early 1960's, when I was managing Boots pharmacy in Uppingham, I had an unnerving experience. I arrived at the shop at about twenty to nine to find the day's delivery of goods was still outside on the pavement and my porter was making no attempt to move the things inside. Something had obviously gone wrong with the delivery that morning.

"Have the goods come late, Reg?" I asked

"No." He shook his head and looked apprehensively into the side entrance.

I could see he was agitated. This was unusual as he was normally a very placid man. I asked "What's wrong?"

Reg peered into the open side door. "I'm not going in there. It's haunted!"

I frowned. "Haunted?"

"Take a look for yourself." He pointed into the dark entrance.

I knew the other staff would soon be arriving and I had to take charge of the suituation so I made my way into the shop. Halfway down the side passage I came to an obstacle. Several cases of Ribena, a red coloured blackcurrant drink, had been tipped onto the floor and some of the glass bottles had broken. The syrup had spread across the white tiles like a large patch of blood. In the centre of this crimson pool were two leather garden gloves placed palms down. They looked just like a pair of outstretched hands. I tiptoed around the sticky patch and continued into the back shop.

As I neared the staff area I could hear running water and there were clouds of steam filling the air. The sound

50

came from the two cloakrooms. When I investigated I found both gas water heaters were turned fully on. Hot water was pouring down the sinks and both rooms were thick with clouds of water vapour. The moisture streaming down the walls and windows, and the amount of steam billowing in the air, suggested the heaters had been running all night!

In the back shop we kept bags of dry drugs on tall wooden shelves. The powders stored on the top shelves had all fallen off and were lying on the floor. There was a regular line of burst bags looking as if someone had deliberately dropped each one into place. It was a total mess! Red, Yellow and Blue ochre, which we sold for raddle, Powdered Chalk, Boracic Ballroom Flake, and the contents of several other split bags lay in a straight row looking like so many exploded bombs. Each bag had burst open and the contents had scattered over the floor.

I turned off the water heaters and opened all the windows to disperse the steam then checked that the back entrance was still secure, but I found no sign of a break in.

I explained to Reg what had happened, then we got the goods in and he set about cleaning up the mess. When I had time to stop and consider the situation I was at a loss to understand it. It seemed obvious that someone had left the hot taps running all night but I had been on rota duty that evening and was the last to leave the shop. I had checked everywhere before I left the premises. There was definitely no tap running in either cloakroom at that time. I decided I must get a plumber to check the hot water taps in case they were faulty but it did seem unlikely they would both malfunction on the same night.

Reg was still convinced there was a supernatural explanation for the events of that morning. This attitude concerned me for you couldn't meet a more level headed man.

My porter was a retired carpenter who also helped the local undertaker deal with funerals and the laying out of bodies. His fears made me feel uneasy but I kept my concerns to myself and concentrated on opening the pharmacy.

With the goods safely in the back shop, I walked into the sales area and the dispensary. When I turned on the lights I got another shock. In the centre of the dispensing bench was a complete ring of dead flies about a foot in diameter. That had certainly not been there the previous evening. When I'd finished the rota duty, I had wiped down the work surface and closed the dispensary as usual. I quickly swept the insects into the bin before the other staff arrived. The business with the running taps and the damaged stock I could just about dismiss as an oversight on my part but a perfect circle of dead flies appearing overnight was far more sinister.

That day was busy in the shop and the events of the morning were soon put to the back of my mind until mid morning when one of the local midwives called in to the pharmacy to refill her medicine bag.

"I need some more Pethilorfan." She produced the signed order for the pethidine injections.

"Keeping you busy are they?" I chatted to her as I filled in the Controlled Drug register.

She nodded, then said "I see you've been working all hours as well."

I looked up from the register in surprise.

The nurse continued. "I saw you in here last night when I drove home at about 1am. Must have been a urgent prescription to call you out at that hour of the morning."

I closed the register. "You saw me here in the middle of the night? What were doing out so late?"

She smiled. "I was driving past after a home delivery in Bisbrooke. The dispensary lights were on and I could see you through the front windows."

I put my pen down and frowned. I had not been called out that night. The shop was securely locked and all in darkness when I left at 7pm, after the evening rota duty.

"Are you sure it was me?"

"It was a figure in a dark suit. I presumed it was you. I didn't actually stop and look closely as I was so late going home."

I just shook my head. This final revelation supported my porter's fears. I am certain something supernatural had happened in the pharmacy that winter's night.

Fortunately nothing of that nature ever happened again while I was working at Uppingham. It was a one off occurrence and a complete mystery.

Chapter Nine - Sheep and the Public School

When I took over the Boots store in Uppingham in the early 1960's, I realised it was an unusual business. Uppingham Public School was one of the main employers in the village and was all pervading. Each school house ran an account with the shop. Uppingham schoolboys would come with written authorities from their house masters and we would charge the items to the house account. At the end of each term I had to itemise each boys purchases and send an account to the house master concerned. It was a system I had not met as a relief manager all over the Midlands area.

On the whole, Uppingham School boys were well mannered and polite but occasionally, as boys can be, I met one who was trouble. I recall a young man who came into the shop asking for a large tin of Sodium Chlorate weed killer but he did not have a written authority for it. Knowing it could be used to make explosives, I refused to sell it to him. The boy went to a local gardening outlet and purchased the item there. He called back at the shop to show me he had obtained some Sodium Chlorate and acted very clever about it.

I was conerned about the incident and contacted his house master who I knew quite well. I warned him what had happened. I was worried the boy might do something silly and start a fire at the school; he certainly had no legitimate use for a large amount of garden weedkiller. His house master thanked me profusely and said he would deal with the problem.

Some weeks later I had a visit from the Boots Area Director bearing a letter complaining about my behaviour in refusing to sell a weedkiller to a genuine customer. The director was very stern with me until I explained to him the customer was a 15 yr old school boy who would probably have burned down the local public school with Boots weedkiller. Needless to say, that instantly change the tone of the meeting.

The same boy came to my notice again some time later when I understand he made himself an electric fire to heat his room. Unfortunately he chose to make it out of a cardboard box and caused a fire in the dormitory! I suppose boys will be boys! He probably grew up to be a gifted scientist.

The system of having goods on account was common in most Boots stores in the 1960s. At Uppingham we had accounts for most of the farmers and many other local people. We had several titled customers who all ran monthly accounts with the store. The farmers, who did not receive a regular wage but made their money only when they sold stock or crops, would understandably only pay once or twice a year. This was a constant bone of contention with Boots head office. Some of the farmers would pay their bill after a year and even ask for a discount! Coming from Lincolnshire, I was used to this tactic and told them I really ought to be charging them interest as they had taken so long to pay what they owed!

One of the first things I realised when I took over Boots store in Uppingham was the need to get up to date with my knowledge of sheep and cattle management. My experience as an apprentice in the fens was heavily biased towards horticulture and my time since then had been spent in town and city shops as a relief manager. My experience covered stores in the Midlands from Newport Pagnell in the South to Ashby in the North, and from Kings Lynn in the East to Rugby in the West of the region. It was a varied experience but tended to be a short stay in each store so time was spent mainly on dispensing and on management duties. When I arrived in Rutland I found there was more grassland farming than South Lincolnshire where I had been apprenticed. The Rutland farmers relied more on sheep and cattle farming. There were some food crops such as cereals, which Boots supplied Cornox and Iso Cornox sprays for, but on the whole the business was different.

Sheep suffer from many problems. They can get attacked by Blow Flies and eaten alive by the maggots; they are prone to foot rot and to parasites such as Mites, Lice and Ticks. The method of controlling the parasites, apart from constant vigilance and good husbandry, was to dip the sheep in a chemical bath to eliminate the causes.

Usually in spring and winter each year the whole flock would be dipped, which involved submerging each animal in a solution to kill the parasites. I had a surprise one morning when the Boots farming rep called at the store and informed me I was responsible for dipping some of the sheep in the area.

"How are you at sheep dipping?" He asked

I looked at him and smiled, expecting to see he was pulling my leg but he looked serious enough. "Sheep dipping? Where do you expect me to do that? The back yard behind the shop is hardly big enough to swing a cat."

"You have a sheep dip at the top of Newtown Road."

That really did take me by surprise. At that time I was still living in Leicester and travelling to Uppingham every day to work while our bungalow was being built so I wasn't familiar with the outskirts of the town. Newtown Road was a small lane near where I would eventually live but I had never been down the road as it only lead to a green lane that eventually joined the main road to Corby. It was almost a dead end.

"Actually we have a shepherd locally who does the dipping for us." The rep explained. "Phillip will do the dipping and make a note of whose sheep he treats and how many are put through. All you need to do is charge the farmers' accounts with the cost. We charge them so much per head."

"I'm surprised they don't dip their own sheep." I had seen mobile sheep dips on some farms in the past.

"The larger farms will do but the smaller flocks don't warrant that cost so the farmers will bring their sheep to our sheep dip and we do it for them."

I was intrigued by this idea. "Do many Boots shops have their own sheep dips? I 've worked across most of the East Midlands and never come across it before."

"No you're almost unique. The only other one I know is up at Leek in Staffordshire."

When the day came for the sheep dipping I went down to see the spectacle for myself. Newtown road was blocked by dozens of farm vehicles and trailers. Hundreds of sheep were coralled on the road awaiting their turns to go though the chemical dip. The farmers helped Phillip handle their flocks putting the sheep through the dip, one at a time at a fast rate. As each sheep entered the tile lined dipping trough its head was thrust under the surface of the solution to ensure all of it was treated. Each flock was rounded up in a fenced off area then loaded back into their trailers and taken back to their farms. It took most of the day to complete the task. After the job was finished Phillip gave me his notebook with all the details of numbers and owners so I could prepare the accounts.

I watched the dipping for some time and was pleased I had bothered to attend as that was the last occasion that Boots Uppingham was to dip sheep. Soon afterwards the land containing the dip was sold and houses were built on it. It was the beginning of my time at that store and the end of an era for sheep dipping by Boots store in Uppingham.

We sold many other products to the sheep farmers. Foot rot sprays and ointment were a regular commodity. Sheep can develop foot rot if they are kept on damp land. The flock was regularly walked through a shallow bath of antiseptic solution and of Copper Sulphate solution. The farmer had to take care this poisonous copper solution was not ingested by the sheep drinking it, so the flock was kept on the move. It was important that sheep with long wool coats did not get the solution on them as it could stain the fleece permanently and discolour it. They also had to ensure non of the solution got onto nursing ewe's teats as their lambs might take it in when they suckled. The farmer had to check for lame animals and pare away the rotten parts of the foot before the animal was put through the foot bath. There were other treatments we sold such as aerosol sprays, ointments and pastes to prevent and treat this condition.

At tupping time, when the ram was put to the ewes to fertilise them, the farmers used coloured preparations so they could keep account of which ewes had been served. We used to stock coloured powders called raddle in three colours; red, yellow and blue. The shepherd would make up this powder into a paste and spread it on the ram's chest so that it would leave a permanent mark on the ewe's back when it was served. The use of different colours allowed the shepherd to know at what time of the year a particular ewe became pregnant, that gave him a good idea of when it would lamb. They staggered the tupping so that the lambing would not all occur in a short period and they used the different colours to tell the times the diffrent groups of ewes would drop their lambs.

Another condition that affected the local farmer stock was Warble Fly attacks in cattle. We sold packets of Warble Fly Dressing, which were made up into solution and painted onto the beasts' backs.

The Ox Warble Fly lays its eggs from May to August each year. It lays the eggs mainly on the hairs of the animal's hind legs. When the eggs hatch out they bore their way into the animal and wander about its system. In the winter months the larvae appear under the skin on the back of the infected animal and will eventually eat their way through the skin causing much damage to that area. Any skin holed in this way produced poor leather.

In those days the only time the farmers could eradicate the maggots was at the stage they bored breathing holes in the skin, prior to leaving the animal. Cattle showing signs of the infestation were treated with Warble Fly dressing at this stage. The dressing, sometimes of Derris or other insecticide, was applied to the backs of the animals with a wire brush or other implement to ensure it got into the maggots' breathing holes in the skin and killed the maggots inside.

Another problem with cattle that I had never met before was the Staggers. When I first met this term I pictured drunken cows staggering about the fields but soon learned the condition was much more serious than that and could actually kill the animals.

The symptoms of this dangerous condition include staggering, restlessness and agressive behaviour in cattle. Cows badly affected may fall down and suffer convulsions or even die. Staggers is caused by low magnesium- Hypomagnesaemia, to give it its scientific name, generally occured in the spring when the cows were producing much milk and were feeding on rapidly growing grass. The treatment was to replace the low level of magnesium in the animals diets. We sold Cattle Licks, which were brick shaped blocks containing magnesium amd calcium salts. These were put into the fields, fixed to fence posts where the cattle could lick them. Magnesium in the form of oxide was sometimes spread onto the grassland as Calcined

Magnesite powder to be ingested with the grass eaten, but in serious cases the only answer was for the animal to be injected with a calcium and magnesium sterile solution. This solution was injected under the skin behind the cow's shoulder and the area massaged to disperse the injection into the tissues; this form of treatment often worked surprisingly quickly.

You will gather from the above details that country chemists in those days were expected to stock and understand a lot about veternary products as well as dispensing for humans and selling over the counter medical products.

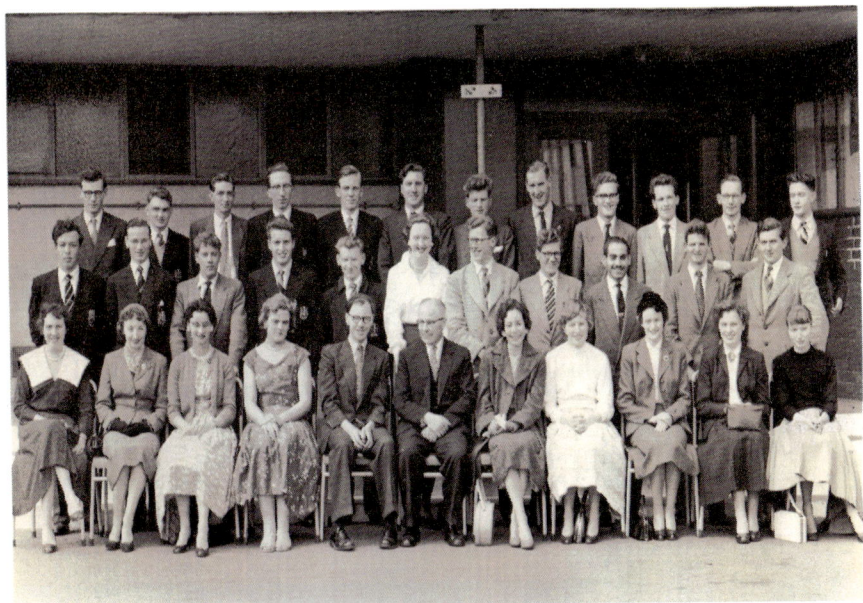

Group photograph of Leicester School of Pharmacy on a visit to May & Baker Ltd on the 28th May 1957. The author is in the middle row, 5th from the left, immediately behind Mr Travers, one of the lecturers. Colin Gunn, head of the department, is seated in the centre front.

Fig 1.

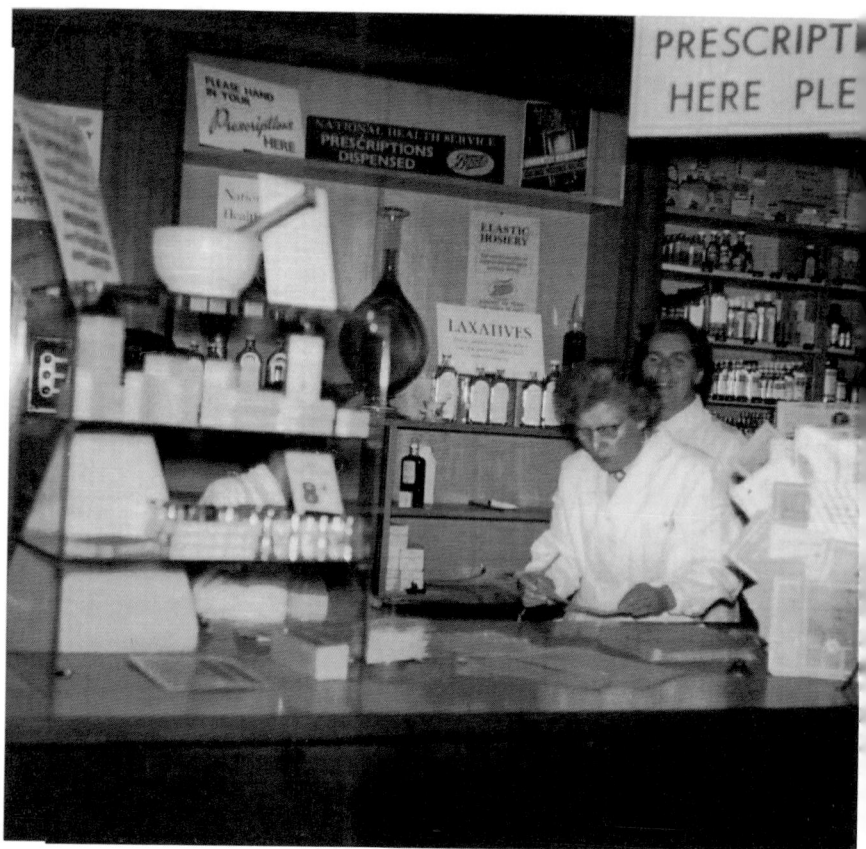

Prescription reception desk at Boots Gallowtree Gate, Leicester in the early 1960s. The lady at the front of the desk was Mrs Black, one of the late night team the author joined after time in the RAMC.

Fig 2.

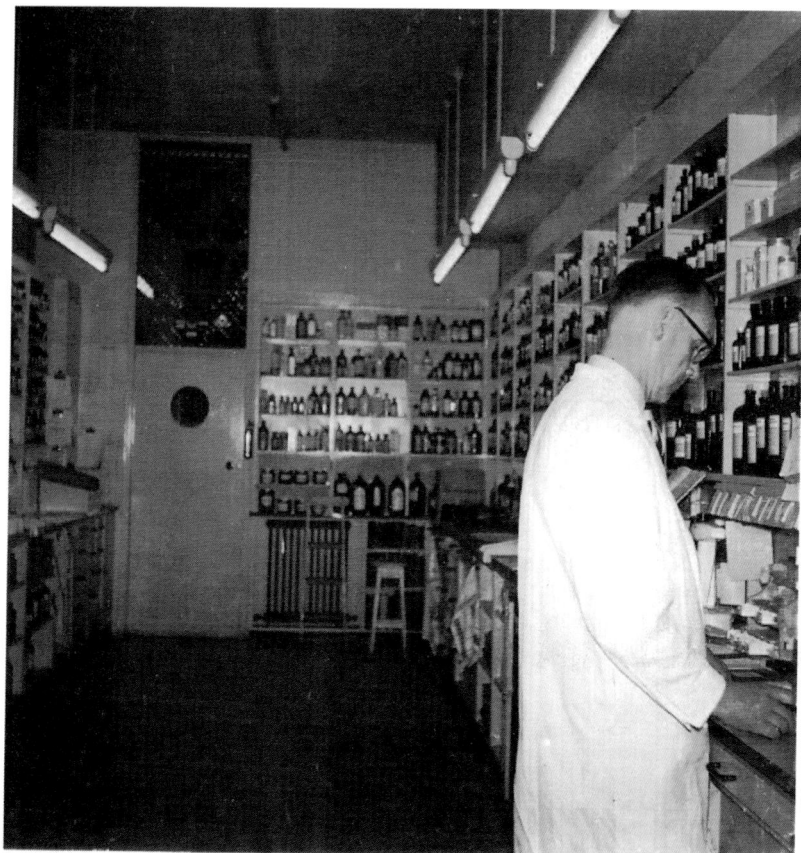

The dispensary at Boots Gallowtree Gate. Arthur Ashley, the dispensary manager is working at the bench. The ready printed labels can be seen in front of him. The shelves are lines with bottles of liquid medicaments used to prepare the many mixtures and liquid medicines in use in the early 1960s.

Fig 3.

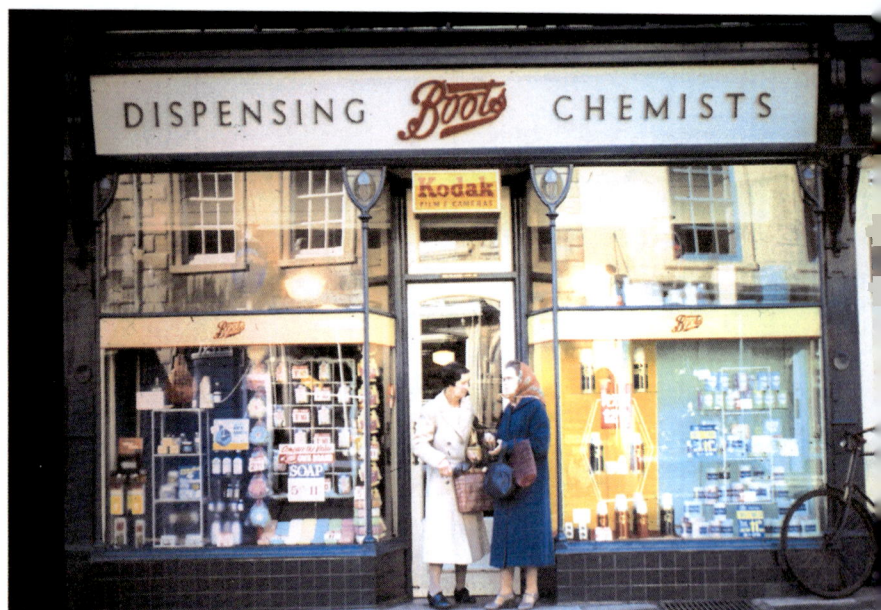

Boots Uppingham store in the early 1960s, when the author took the shop over as manager.

Fig 4.

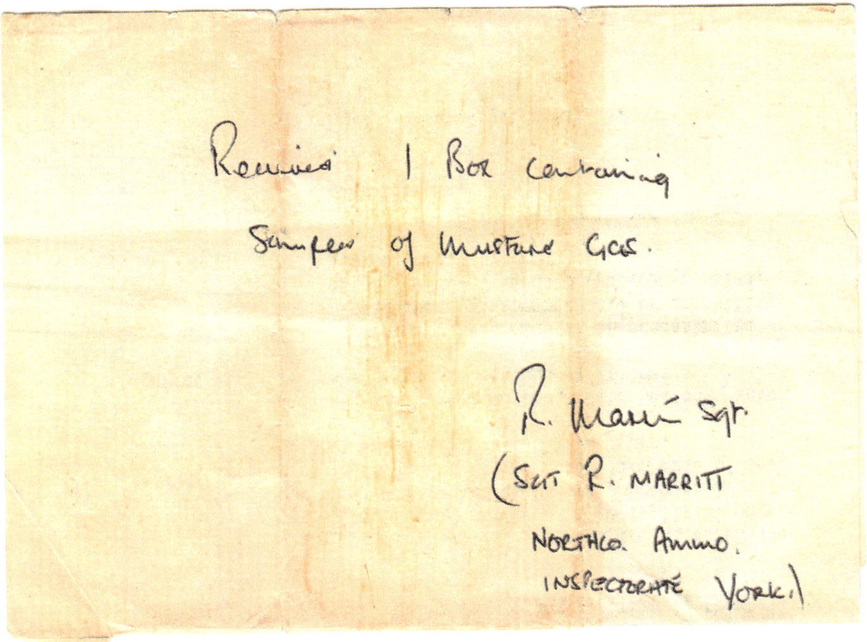

Received 1 Box containing
Samples of Mustard Gas.

R. Marri Sgt.
(SGT R. MARRITT
NORTH Co. AMMO.
INSPECTORATE YORK.)

The receipt given for the Mustard Gas.

Fig 5.

WAR GAS SAMPLES.

INSTRUCTIONS FOR USE.

1. The war gas samples contained in this box are supplied for the exclusive use of Public Analysts and must not under any circumstances be handled by unauthorised persons. The box should be stored in a safe place when not in use.

2. The contents of the box comprise:

   1 bottle with sealed-in dropping-rod containing 1cc. of liquid mustard gas (labelled M).

   1 bottle as above, containing 1cc. of liquid lewisite (labelled L).

   Each bottle is packed in charcoal in a sealed tin, bearing the letter M or L on its lid.

3. Protective gloves should be worn on each and every occasion on which the contents of the box are handled, and should be decontaminated immediately after use by immersion in boiling water for 30 minutes. If protective gloves are not available, the hands should be well scrubbed with soap and hot water at frequent intervals.

4. After removal of the tins from the box, the soldered strips securing the lids should be ripped off, and the tins opened in a well-ventilated fume-cupboard. The adhesive tape securing the stoppers of the bottles on issue should be carefully removed and destroyed by burning, but the absorbent charcoal surrounding the bottles should, as far as possible, be left in position. The bottles should not be removed from the tins or handled unnecessarily, and great care must be exercised in opening them and securely stoppering them after use.

5. The liquid gases should only be removed from the bottles in very small quantities by means of the dropping rods attached to the stoppers, and care should be taken not to allow liquid to come into contact with the neck of the bottle. If this should occur, the neck should be wiped out with dry filter paper before replacing the stopper, and the filter paper burned or treated as in 7.

6. If a drop of liquid gas accidentally falls on to the bench etc. during transference, the liquid should be immediately wiped up with a dry cotton wool swab (which should be subsequently burned, or treated as in 7) and the contamination area of the bench covered with bleach-water paste for 24 hours.

7. Immediately after use, all apparatus etc, which has come into contact with the gases should be cleaned as follows:

   Mustard gas:-   Immerse for 5-10 minutes in concentrated
                    nitric acid (glassware etc.) or in boiling
                    water for 20-30 minutes (rubber articles,
                    gloves, etc.)

   Lewisite:-   Immerse for 5-10 minutes in 15% aqueous
                    caustic soda.

J. W. TOWERS & CO. LTD.,   WIDNES.

Mustard Gas leaflet   Fig 6.

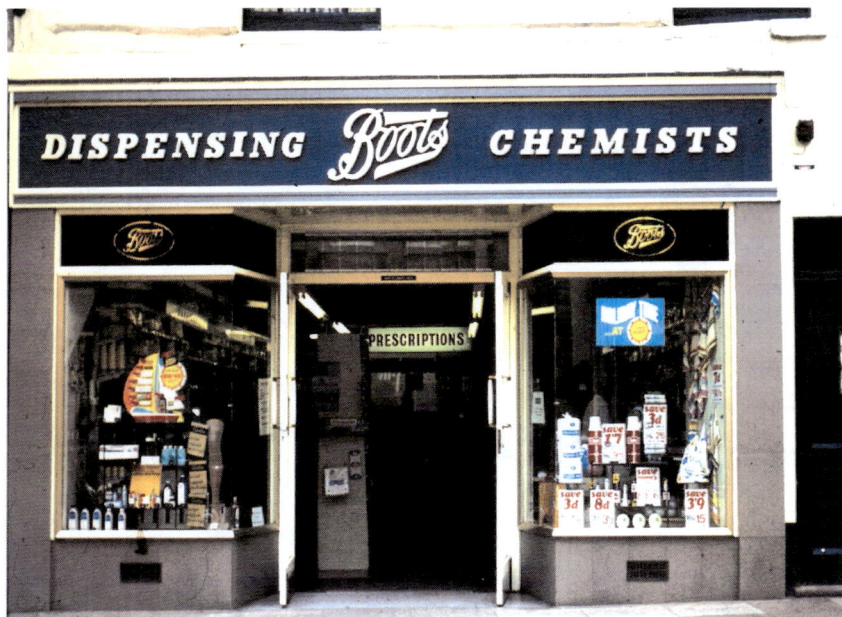

Boots Uppingham after the refit in the 1960s.

Fig 7.

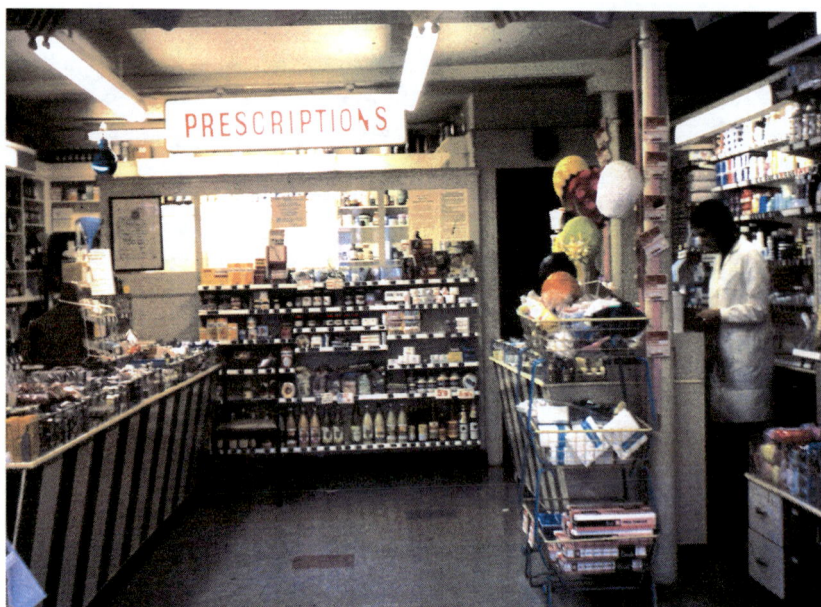

The sales area of Boots Uppingham after the refit in the late 1960s.

Fig 8

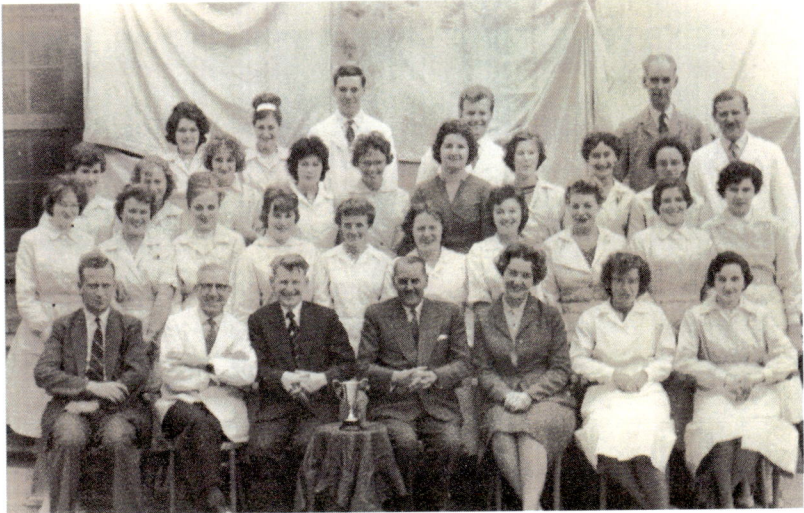

Staff of Boots Rugby when they won the cup for the best business results in Territory 2 in the late 1950s. The author took charge of this store for some time when the manager, Mr F H Williams, was seriously ill. Frank Williams is seated at the front to the right of the cup on this photograph.. The author is seated at his side.

Fig 9.

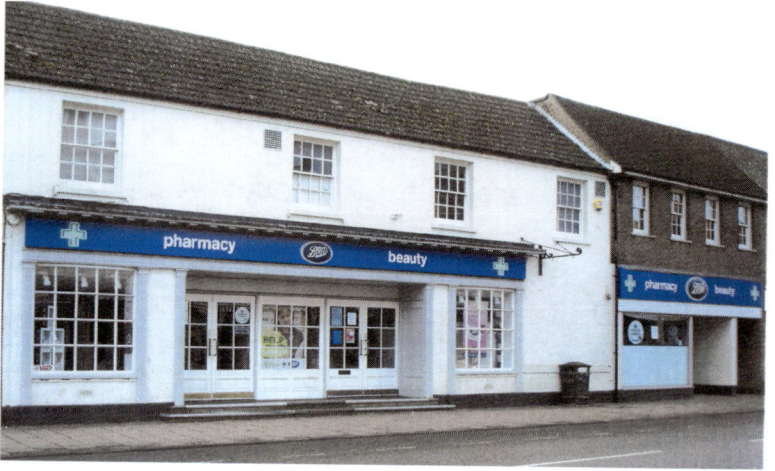

Boots store in Oakham

Fig 10.

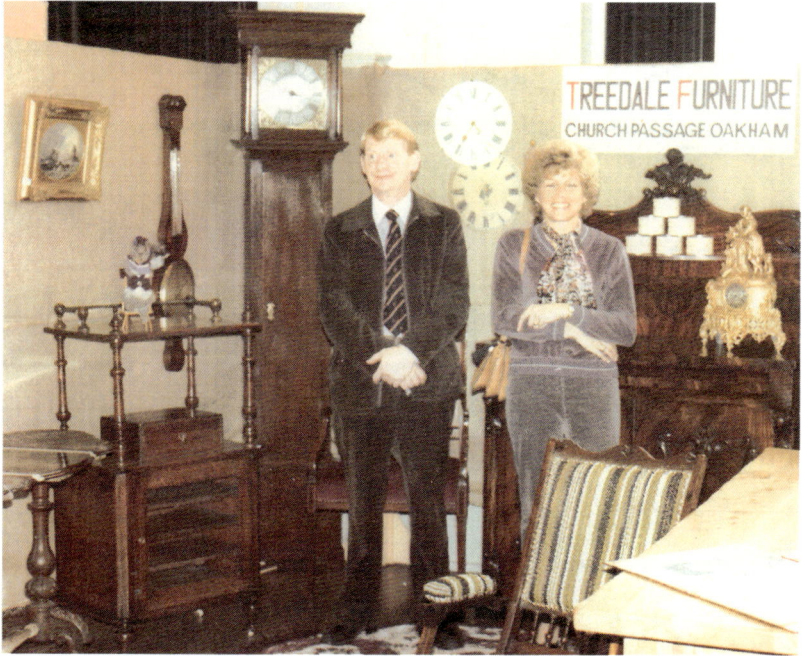

The author and his late wife manning an Antique Fair stand at the Victoria Hall in Oakham in the 1970s . His clocks and barometers were displayed at Treedale Antiques at that time.

Fig 11.

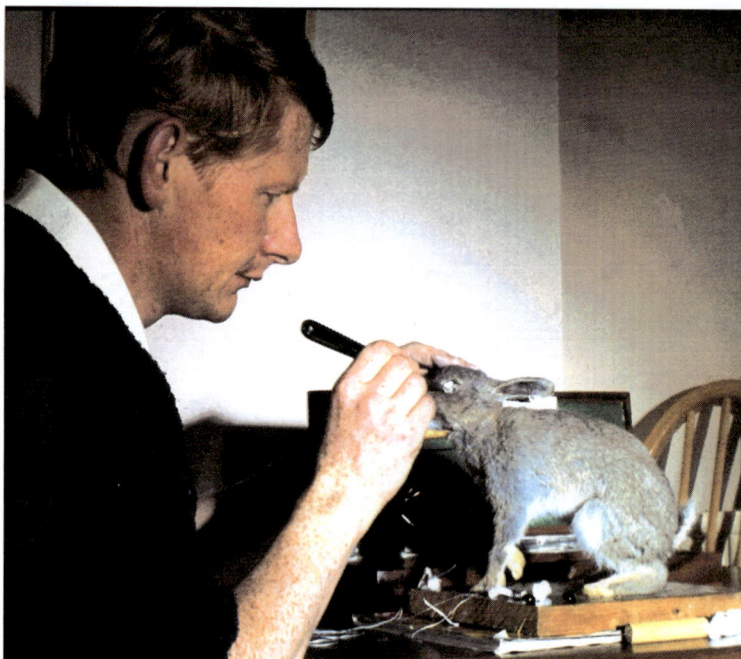

The author setting up a rabbit for the forestry commission.
to take to the East of England Show

Fig 12

Chapter Ten - Taxidermy & Clocks at Uppingham.

In spite of my long hours at the pharmacy in Uppingham, I took up my hobby of taxidermy again once I had settled into the job. I partitioned off the end of my garage and set up a studio there. As a schoolboy I had helped the taxidermist at the Spalding Bird Museum and had been taught the craft by him. I was always interested in wildlife and biology so the hobby fitted me well. In a country area like Uppingham, I soon got known for something as unusual as taxidermy. Slowly I began to do work for the local farmers. Many Fox Masks on shields and game birds were set up and sold as commissions.

Uppingham at that time was a keen fox hunting area being covered by the locally based Cottesmore Hunt. This lead to some interesting circumstances. It was frowned upon for tennant farmers to kill foxes on their land, even if the foxes were killing lambs and causing some loss to them. The Hunt preferred the foxes to be available for a day's sport. Because of these circumstances I would frequently get a secret phone call late in the evening.

"Is that the taxidermist? Would you like a fox to stuff?" It was usually an anonymous caller and struck me at first as very unusual, until I soon realised what was going on.

"Yes. What can I do for you?"

"There's a dead fox in a sack at the roadside ..." The locality was usually out in the countryside well away from any villages. "If you would like it you can have it. It'll save me burying it."

I would thank the donor and go after dark to pick up the carcass. Once the Foxes were skinned and set up there was a ready market for them. If the carcass was too damaged I would usually just set up the mask and brush on a decorative shield. I sometimes sold these through local antique shops.

On one occasion I received a call informing me there were two young fox cubs dead on the road just outside Uppingham. The fox family had been crossing the main road at night and had been hit by a passing lorry. The carcasses were on the grass verge. I set the pair of cubs play fighting each other as they are frequently seen doing in the wild. Those cubs were set up and cased and are still displayed in one of the local farm houses.

Fish were also favourite specimens to be stuffed. We are well served with fishing lakes in Rutland. Recently, they made the Rutland Water reservoir and there was already the much smaller but older Eyebrook Reservoir near Stoke Dry village. Both provide fly fishing of a high order. One of my favourite fish to set up and case was the Brown Trout but there tended to be more Rainbow Trout brought to me. Rainbow Trout are a very colourful fish but I personally find the Brown Trout more attractive looking.

If the specimen was a good large one, the fisherman usually wanted it set up in a case with a glass front. Sometimes they even went to the expense of a bow fronted case, which made a splendid trophy. I would set the fish in a realistic riverbed setting and signwrite the name of the fisherman, the weight of the fish, the date and place caught, in gold leaf lettering inside the glass front. Occasionally I would be asked to set up a Deer head or Salmon, which were sent down from Scotland.

As the wild Mink became a problem, more farmers trapped them. Rutland suffered from these introductions, which had been released from Mink farms by animal rights protesters with no inkling of the damage such predators could do to the local wildlife. Some of the Mink were brought to me to be set up. They made a very acceptable specimen.　　One particular Mink was sent to me from Northern Ireland. It was sent by areoplane, frozen and well packed in insulating material. The specimen was a large one with an interesting story.

The Irish Mink had been attacking the chickens kept by a British Army Major, stationed in Northern Ireland at the time He had shot it with an air pistol and hit it straight between the eyes. He was obviously a very accomplished shot. That one was cased and returned by air, the same way it had come to me. My hobby lead to me giving talks on the subject to interested groups such as the Rutland Natural History Society, Young Farmers Groups and other Natural History Societies in the area.

I advertised in the Yellow Pages at one time to get more business for my hobby and had some extremely unusual requests. I do recall being asked if I would stuff a giant crocodile! The circumstances were bizzare. A travelling circus had a very large live crocodile, which they displayed in a transparent tank to the paying public. It had died. They telephoned me one evening.

"Can you stuff a crocodile for us?"

I had never set up such a large reptile so I was cautious. "How big is it?"

The owner was very proud of his specimen. "It's the largest in captivity in the British Isle. It's about 25 feet long from nose to tail."

"How long has it been dead?" I had visons of a very large smelly carcass.

"We don't know. We just found it dead in its tank."

That was all I wanted to hear. "I'm afraid my studio is far too small to handle anything that size. Sorry I can't help you." The man was disappointed but there was no way I could handle such a large specimen even if I had wanted the commission. I was happy ticking over setting up small mammals such as foxes, and badgers, which were road kills, and dead birds such as Owls, picked up by the locals from the roadsides.

Another problem of scale happened a few years later. I was contacted by a Whisky distillery in Scotland that wanted to supply each of their retail outlets with a stuffed Grouse, which would advertise their brand of Whisky. We corresponded for some time and I eventually realised they wanted one thousand Grouse set up in exactly the same pose, to be used as counter displays. This was a large order but I reasoned it would pay well and I could supply the specimens over a period of months. The problem came when I asked the firm to send me the first batch of dead birds, then I was informed they expected me to supply the birds as well as set them up! Needless to say there were no Grouse available in Rutland and I had no intention of spending my life shooting up in Scotland, so the deal fell through.

As well as my taxidermy hobby I developed an interest in grandfather clocks while I was living in Uppingham. I was on the look out for a grandfather clock movement and dial because I wanted the challenge of building a wooden clock case, and I just fancied a longcase clock standing in my home.

In Uppingham market place at that time was an antique shop run by John Tasker who was a member of the British Antique Dealers Association. John was a knowledgeable antique dealer and a good friend. He sold me a basket case of a grandfather clock, which I bought just for the works and face. I took the clock home in several pieces intending to salvage the works and dial and throw away the pieces of the broken oak case. When I explained this to John, he assured me the case was more valuable than the works, even in its broken state. This did seem odd to me but he explained that wooden cases rot and get wood worm so they are rarer than the brass works or Iron dials. This set me thinking and I decided to restore the old case as well as the works and dial and keep them together.

My abiding interest in antique clocks dates back to that project and lead to me restoring many longcase and other old clocks over the years. When the locals knew about my interest, I was often requested to repair a clock or set up a grandfather clock that refused to run after someone had moved home.

I recall one family who asked me on several occasions to call and get their clock going. This was unusual as once set up properly, grandfather clocks go on ticking and telling the time for years. After three such calls I decided to do some detective work to ascertain the problem. It transpired the lady of the house had a cleaning lady who regularly moved the clock to vacuum clean the carpet under it! Once I explained she must not move it every few weeks, the problem stopped.

My interest in clocks eventually lead to requests to restore Mercury Barometers, which was a service I also offered. All of these hobbies, as well as the chemist business, put me in regular touch with the locals and made the job very fulfilling.

Chapter Eleven - The Winter of 1963

The winter of 1963 was a particularly cold one with snow and ice over much of the country. In the East Midlands, in Rutland, where I was managing Boots Uppingham pharmacy, we were sometimes cut off completely because of the hills in and out of the village. There was a steep slope into Uppingham whichever way you approached it; from Corby to the South, Oakham to the North, Gasworks Hill to the East and Wardley Hill to the West. There was no bypass on the A47 in those days and all the traffic came through the village. Because of these steep inclines the roads soon became impassable, blocked by stranded cars and lorries, which had skidded out of control. That winter had been a hard one. Customers from outlying hamlets such as Bisbrooke, Seaton and Ridlington regularly avoided the roads and came to the village across the fields by tractor to pick up their groceries and their prescriptions. There was an occasion when one of the local doctors drove into Bisbrook, a nearby village, to treat a patient. The ambulance was called and took the patient into hospital but the doctor, who had forgotten his tyre chains, was stranded in the village until a local garage rescued him.

Boots was the only pharmacy in Uppingham at that time and as the only pharmacist I was on call around the clock for emergency medicines and other essential chemist supplies. The shop was open from 9am until 6pm then I undertook dispensing duty until 7pm. On the half day, which was on a Thursday, we closed the shop at 1pm but I went back from 6pm to 7pm to do the dispensing duty. Sundays and every bank holiday I did a dispensing duty from 12 noon to 1pm.

66

On Christmas Eve, I closed the shop at 7pm and walked home through the deepening snow, pleased to be finished for the day. I had officially finished work until mid-day on Christmas day when I was due to do an hours dispensing duty.

After I had had my evening meal and was sitting with my wife in front of a roaring fire, we had an unexpected phone call. It was from the Rutland Police. "Is that Mr Merchant the Uppingham pharmacist?"

"Yes."

"This is the police station in Oakham. We urgently need you to open the Uppingham pharmacy."

That was a very unusual request. If there was an out of hours call for a prescription it was invariably the local doctors who telephoned me. I queried the caller.

"What's the problem?"

"We need baby milk, feeding bottles and other items to look after several babies. We also need some urgent supplies of medicines. We have several families stranded overnight in your village."

I was surprised at this request but realised it must indeed be urgent for them to ring me on such a terrible night. I knew I had to go and open the shop again.

"I'll be down as soon as I can make it."

"Thank you, Sir. The local officers will be parked outside the shop waiting for you"

I explained the call to my wife, who was as amazed as I was at this turn of events. She parted the curtains at our front window and looked out at Stockerston Crescent where we lived. "It's blowing a gale and snowing even harder. It must be knee deep by now and drifting even deeper. You'd better be extra careful walking down the hill to the shop. There's no way you can take the car."

I took a look outside and agreed with her. Large

snowflakes were billowing past the street lights completely obscuring the view across the street. Suddenly I had an idea. "I'll ski down, love."

I had made myself some cross country skis from straight grained Ash that same autumn with the help of Teddy Toon, the local undertaker and a fine cabinet maker. Teddy had an electric plane and a steamer to shape the skis. I had fitted my skis with telemark bindings, which I made from aircraft grade aluminium sheet and leather straps. That winter I had learned how to use them by trudging up and skiing down Castle Hill in the snow on my days off. This was an opportunity to use them properly.

I put on warm waterproof clothes and skied down to the High Street from where we lived at the top of Stockerston hill on the outskirts of the village. When I got to the shop I found the police car waiting for me. I opened the pharmacy, switched on all the lights and let them in. The officers had some strangers with them who had long lists of the supplies they needed.

"What's going on?" I enquired from one of the policemen who was a local man that I recognised.

"Uppingham is cut off by the snow and ice. We have over forty people stuck in the village who were passing through on their way to spend Christmas with families. We've been rescuing them and bringing them into the village. They can't get anywhere else tonight."

I frowned. "What are you doing with them?"

"Mrs Flood, the manageress of the local cinema, has agreed to open it for the night. She's left the lights on and the heating. They are all camped in there, sitting and lying on the padded seats. They are all warm and dry but there are several mothers with babies with no supplies and at least one man in urgent need of his medicines."

"What about food and drink?" I asked

"We've sorted that out. The Christmas Eve Ball in

Oakham has been cancelled because of the atrocious weather. We've collected all the food t ey'd prepared ready for the interval and have brought it over here by tractor. At least it wont go to waste."

It seemed the police had it all under control.

I collected cartons of baby milk, feeding bottles, tins of baby food, disposable nappies, cough mixtures, paracetamol syrup and other essential items and sold them to the people, then I asked about the prescriptions.

"Hang on I'll get the gentleman." The officer went out to his car.

An elderly man came into the shop and explained he was diabetic and hadn't any insulin with him. He also needed his heart tablets. After some questioning to ascertain which insulin he was using, I managed to do an emergency supply of the injection and supply him with a syringe and the other items he would need. He was lucky we stocked that type of insulin as there were so many different ones. His heart tablets were the usual Digoxin so it was no problem to do an emergency supply.

It took me about an hour to sort out all those people. After I'd closed the shop and made it secure, I strapped on my skis and trudge back up the hill to home.

Next morning, Christmas morning, they had managed to clear the roads enough to get the stranded travellers on their way. By the time I opened the shop at mid-day, they were all continuing on their journeys home or to their families for Christmas.

Gladys Flood, the cinema manageress, called into the pharmacy on her way home from locking up the picture house and wished me a Happy Christmas.

"Have a good Christmas." She said. "It's a good job you and I were available last night."

The vicar also called in on his way to church. "Happy Christmas. I think you and I are the only people working in Uppingham this winter morning." He also thanked me for turning out the previous night; he had visited the cinema earlier that morning after midnight mass to check if all was well.

The rest of the dispensing duty was very quiet, hardly anyone was about that snowy morning. It had been a most unusual Christmas but a satisfying one for all of us.

Chapter Twelve - A Move to Oakham

After several years running Boots in Uppingham and several attempts by Boots to get me to leave the small shop and take on a larger store, I decided I would move. I suppose it was a decision taken partly out of boredom as I needed a new challenge. My daughters were at the stage where a move would not disrupt their education, so I suggested to my district manager that I would like to be considered for the management of Boots shop in Oakham as the incumbent manager was due to retire. At that time managers' names were put forwad for promotion by head office; it was not normal for a manager to suggest a move he fancied. Fortunately, Bob Brown, my territorial manager, was fully behind me and backed my application.

"Just don't let me down as I'm putting my neck on the line for you," was his only comment. He needn't have worried. Boots Oakham did very well under my management, being extended and refitted three times during my years in charge.

Oakham Boots was very different from my previous experience in Uppingham. It was a bigger store with a larger dispensing business than the Uppingham branch and had far more staff. My time was taken up more with management and by the dispensary. I continued my practice of getting to know my customers well, as that meant I could give them a more personal service. Chemists have a unique opportunity to know their regular customers by name as the prescriptions presented to them have the patient's details written on them; that makes it much easier to put a name to a face. The Boots store in Oakham was very succesful, which meant it was refitted and enlarged three times during my tenure as manager.

The final refit took in the next door premises of Dewhurst the butchers when they closed their shops. I was approached to take a promotion and move to an even larger store on a few occasions but as my daughters were growing up and settled at excellent schools in Rutland, I passed over the opportunities and stayed at the Oakham store. In the1970 Boots ceased trading in Farms and Gardens products and concentrated on their core offering of Health and Beauty with some Photographic business, as was traditional with chemists. My main occupation was then even more concentrated on the dispensing and the management side of the business.

Dispensing had also changed radically over the years. Almost all the items supplied were in solid dose forms such as tablets or capsules The few liquid preparations used were supplied ready made and prepacked. Occasionally an unusual item would be ordered and had to be made, but because of product testing regulations, pharmacies ordered these items from Specials Manufacturing Laboratories. Needless to say, they were much more expensive to produce that way but the National Health Service paid for them.

On a few occasions one of the older doctors would order an old preparations, which was not freely available, and I would make it in the dispensary, as we used to in times gone by, but time and regulations did not permit this happening often. One of the older preparations I do recall making was Glycerine of Borax. This product used to be used for some mouth problems and was sold over the counter but it fell into disuse because it was toxic if used in excess. In the past it had a reputation for treating teething problems in infants but that was no longer recommended as Borax could be toxic to babies.

A doctor telephoned me and asked me to get him some of the preparation for a terminally ill patient with a

72

mouth infection No one listed it any more so I turned up the formula in Martindale, the 'Bible' for pharmaceutical knowledge, and made a small jar to complete the prescription. Such requests were few and far between but I did enjoy making them when the occasion presented itself.

During the winter of 1978/79 the country experienced the 'Winter of Discontent.' This was a difficult period in British history when the Trade Unions went on strike. Their industrial action was against the Labour Government's freeze on wages, which Jim Callaghan had instigated. One of the results of this industrial action was the rationing of electricity, which coincided with the dark winter days and nights and with one of the coldest winters for the previous 16 years; not since the awful winter of 1963. The country experienced deep snow and blizzards during the early part of 1979, which made matters worse.

The power supply was cut off for specific areas of the country for fixed times of the day and night to ration what small supplies were available. At home we were fortunate in having fitted a Dragon multifuel stove, which had a flat top where pans and a kettle could be heated. Boiling the water, heating liquids such as soup and making toast by opening the burner doors, ensured we had hot meals. The experience took me back to my boyhood when we would regularly toast bread on a long fork held over an open fire. The Dragon also kept the living room warm and heated the water in the storage tank so we were relatively well served. I had also collected a few Victorian oil lamps, which were decorative but useful in times of emergency. In some ways the log fire and the warm glow of oil lamps looked romantic and were a nice reminder of an earlier era but the strikes were inconveneint and especially so for businesses. Most of the local shops closed during the blackout periods but as Chemists we had little choice but to try to give an emergency service. The townsfolk coped as best they could with this inconvenience. All the shops soon ran out of candles and hot water bottles as the dark and cold took hold.

At the Oakham branch of Boots the Chemist we tried hard to keep a service going to help our customers. We kept the dispensary and the medical section of the shop open in spite of it being too dark to see and in spite of it being very cold. I brought some oil lamps into the store from home to light the dispensary and we blocked off the sections of the shop that were not absolutely necessary; it was essential to stop customers wandering about in the dark and possibly harming themselves. Staff members worked in their coats and warm clothes using battery operated torches to find the goods for the customers. Regulations stated that the store should be at a reasonable temperature for work but all my staff volunteered to help even though they could have objected. As the electric tills would not work, we made lists of the sales in a notebook and put the items and cash through the tills when we had the electricity supply back on again.

In Oakham High Street at the time, we had a local Electricity Board shop where they displayed a list of times when we could expect the electricity to be turned on. It was a daily task to send a member of staff to that shop to take a note of the times we could expect to have power and when we would have to cope with no power. In the dispensary we had to revert to hand written labels as the computer labellers were not working. It was a sobering thought that my predecessors as apothecaries regularly worked like that by flickering candle light when the daylight failed.

People soon took to shopping during the switched on periods and only came into the store for emergencies, such as medicines and prescriptions, when we were in darkness. This was not surprising as the street lights were also affected and parts of the town were regularly in darkness.

Today it would be impossible to carry on dispensing without an electricity supply to the computers but we found a way during that difficult period to satisfy our customers and supply their medicines. After this experience, Boots supplied the shop with a small petrol driven generator, which could produce enough electricity to keep a few emergency lights on.

One other unusual incident sticks in my memory from my days at Oakham. We were a busy dispensary and took it in turns with the other Chemist shop in town to give a dispensing rota duty. When it was our turn, I was on duty alternate weeks until 7pm on week nights and for an hour at mid-day on the Sundays and Bank Holidays. We only opened the store to dispense prescriptions and to sell medical items. There was also an emergency out of hours service, which I joined, to supply urgently needed items such as Oxygen and prescriptions at any hour of the day or night. This was accessed by telephone calls from the doctors or occasionally the local police.

The occasion I especially remember was one Christmas when I was on dispensing duty and there was an Influenza epidemic in the area. Usually on rota I would dispense perhaps five or six prescriptions but on this occasion the demand was phenominal! I had not asked my dispenser to cover the rota duty with me as I expected it to be very quiet being Christmas Day, but I was mistaken.

In the event, I kept the pharmacy open for three hours and dispensed over 200 prescriptions that Bank Holiday. Doctor Woolford was on duty at the local medical practice and all the local prescriptions were issued by him. I had a prescription query and telephoned the surgery to get the duty doctors home number so I could contact him. I was very surprised when the doctor himself answered the telephone.

"What's going on? Are you open at the surgery?" I asked him.

"It's so busy I have opened the surgery and am sitting at my desk dealing with patients' needs as they ring in. There's no way I could cope with home visits on this scale."

I sorted out the query with him, wished him a Happy Christmas and got on with the backlog of prescriptions facing me on the dispensary bench.

When we opened after the holiday period, it took some time to sort out the mess in the shop. Customers who had been queuing for their prescriptions, had picked up other items they wished to buy but realising I was far too busy with the prescriptions to serve them, they had dumped them on the counter or on top of other displays. That was the busiest I have ever been, single handed, on a rota duty.

Chapter Thirteen - Taxidermy & Clocks at Oakham

When I left Uppingham to take over Boots Oakham store I decided to move from my bungalow in Uppingham to a house in Oakham. Many of my friends assumed I would stay living in Uppingham and travel each day but I realised being a Pharmacist on call and doing long hours because of rota duties, would mean I would see little of my family if I stayed living where I was. We sold our bungalow in Uppingham and moved to a house on Cricket Lawns in Oakham, which was within easy walking distance of the store.

I continued with my hobbies of clock restoration and taxidermy once I had completed the move and the necessary alterations to the new home. I had a double garage on Cricket Lawns and made part of that into an outside workshop.

About this period I was approached by the Forestry Commision to set up some specimens for them. They frequently came across dead animals and birds and wanted a small collection to take with them when they gave talks to schools and other interested groups. I had set up a few Grey Squirells and a Heron for them in the past but this time they approached me to set up several animals and birds for a diorama they intended to take to the East of England Show, which was held annually at Peterborough. They wanted to advertise the services they gave.

Specimens of Rabbits, Squirells and woodland birds like Jays, Magpies, Partridges and Pheasants kept arriving at the workshop by the sack load. They even produce a dead Muntjac Deer for me to stuff.

I supplied all of these specimens with no bases, just with their support wires sticking out from the base of their feet, so the forestry workers could fix them exactly where they needed them. They set up a woodland scene at the show and put the specimens into it. I understand it was a great success though I didn't get time to go over and see it. Prince Charles visited the Show that year and commented favourably on the Forestry display. They gave him my business card but I never heard any more from him. It would have been nice to claim Taxidermist by Royal Appointment! On the last day of the Show the exhibitors were surprised by a sudden downpour of rain. The soaking wet specimens were all brought back to my workshop to be dried out and restored; not a task I looked forward to doing.

While I lived on Cricket Lawns I had a telephone call from a local city museum who had been given the carcass of an adult Giraffe that had died in a local Zoo. They wanted it set up to add to their taxidermy collection. I explained to my surprised wife what was needed; she was incredulous that I might even contemplate such a large job.

"Where will you do it?" She asked. "Surely the garage workshop isn't tall enough to accomodate a fully grown Giraffe?"

I had no intention of taking on the commission as it was a job for a team of workers being so large a specimen but I decided to kid her along.

"I think I will do it in the hall. I can stretch the neck up the stairs and fit it in like that. The body and legs can stay downstairs" Unfortunately I couldn't keep up the pretence; she must have detected the twinkle in my eyes.

She just laughed and sighed with relief. I telephoned the museum and told them that reluctantly I hadn't the time or space to do the job for them

After a few years on Cricket Lawns my wife and I decided we would prefer an older property with more room

78

and more facilities. We managed to buy a run down Victorian property on the other side of Oakham; a house with outbuildings and room to expand where I could set up my workshop once again. We set about restoring the house on West Road as a shared project. It made a marvellous family home for us and the children.

Rutland Water was developed during my years at the Oakham store and many more fish were also brought to me to be set up. The local police would also bring me dead Badgers that had been killed on the roads in the area.

One afternoon when I was on a day off I had a telephone call from a firm in Leicester.

"Hello, Is that the taxidermist? This is the Fox's Glacier Mint factory near Leicester. We need someone to repair one of our advertising exhibits."

I was intrigued and enquired what exactly they needed doing.

"We have a stuffed Polar Bear, which we take to exhibitions to advertise our Fox's Glacier Mints. Unfortunately, some children swung on its head the last time we were out and it has a broken neck. Can you repair it for us."

I asked where the specimen was stored and was pleased to find it was just the other side of Leicester, so I made arangements to go over to see the damage.

My wife and I drove over to the factory one afternoon and asked to see the Bear. It was stored in the top of a large warehouse on a high gantry. When I actually saw the Polar Bear close up, I could see the extent of the damage. I realised the skin would have to be removed from the specimen and a new wooden neck made. It was not a job that could be done on site. The other thing I realised was the gigantic size of the Bear- it was over six feet wide and very long - would make it impossible to fit it into my workshop. I decided to kid my wife once again that I might consider the job

"We could load it onto the roof rack of the car to get it home, Love. Imagine the heads that will turn when we drive through the centre of Leicester with a giant Polar Bear strapped on top of the car."

Needles to say, she was not fooled. I had to tell the customer there was no way I could cope with such a large specimen. I recommended one of the London taxidermy studios, who had probably stuffed the Bear in the first place.

There came a stage when I was getting too busy with taxidermy and was faced with a choice of carrying on as a Pharmacist or taking up the taxidermy full time. I chose my first love and remained a Chemist, cutting back drastically on any taxidermy work I chose to take on. I did give the ocassional talk on the subject to local Natural History groups with the aid of a set of colured slides I made of the processes involved, but I chose to only do taxidermy work that really interested me.

I was also becoming more interested in Creative Writing and Publishing as a hobby and decided to put my taxidermy experience to better use by writing several textbooks on the subject. The books did well and are still in print. When asked if I did taxidermy any more I would say "No but I write about it. It's a much easier and less messy aspect of the craft."

The clock restoration was a different matter. That hobby I found more enjoyable than taxidermy. I could take months restoring a clock and enjoy it when I found time to work on it, in contrast to the taxidermy, which deals with perishable items: once started a taxidermy job must be completed as quickly as possible no matter how long it takes. I continued working on antique clocks for local people and bought some in need of restoration at auction, at the right price, to restore and sell on.

Restored grandfather clocks sold well at that time. I had an arrangement with one or two local antique businesses who would display my clocks and sell them on commission. Occasionally I would sell a longcased clock to one of the foreign airforce officers who were stationed at RAF Cottesmore. They would take them back with them when they were returning to Germany. On the continent British antique longcased clocks were making even better money than they were over here.

Some clocks I put back into antique sales to sell at auction. I just enjoyed the practical work of making and restoring the mechanisms and rebuilding the wooden cases. Pharmacy had been a practical career in my early days when chemists made ointment, creams, mixtures, drops etc. I had even been called upon to make suppositories and individually wrapped powders to complete prescriptions, but dispensing was fast becoming a matter of counting tablets and labelling them. Of course, a pharmacist used his knowledge of medicines to check every prescription for correctness, for dosage, compatibility, and suitability for the patient; he also advised them how to use their medicines correctly. Pharmacist advised customers about over the counter medical products, but the job was becoming less interesting to a practical minded person like myself. I had lived and work through a time of great change for the pharmacy and medical professions; retail pharmacists, in particular, seemed to me to be searching for their place in the new scheme of things. I continued to buy and restore antique clocks as I felt a practical hobby was a necessary change for me from the pressures of business and dispensing, which had become less and less hands on.

My wife and I sold small antiques, such as dolls and jewellery, and restored clocks and barometers, through one or two outlets in Oakham. One of these clocks unfortunately gave me my one and only brush with the law!

I used to take a trip out on my day off and do the rounds visiting antique dealer friends in Northamptonshire, looking for damaged clocks that I could enjoy restoring. I usually bought grandfather clocks as that was my first love but on one occasion I purchased an Edwardian bracket clock, which chimed and struck on the hour. It was an elegant mahogany veneered case with a typical Edwardian floral inlay - a style referred to as Edwardian Sheraton.

The clock had been a presentation piece. This was obvious by the screw holes in the front of it where an engraved plate had been removed.

I restored the clock and offered it for sale in a local antique shop in the Church Passage in Oakham where it was spotted by an Oakham schoolboy.

The boy recognised the clock as one stolen from his grandfather who lived in Northamptonshire. He rightly reported the fact to the police.

My first inkling of a problem was when two detectives approached me in the dispensary at work and asked me if the bracket clock was indeed my property. I confirmed it was and explained where I had obtained it and what had occured since the purchase. They told me it was stolen property and they had confiscated it.

Later that day I spoke to the antique dealer who ran the Church Passage shop. He had been approached and dealt with far less politely than I had experienced! He had told the police the clock was my property and nothing to do with him.

I made a statement telling the police where and when I had bought the clock and any other details I could remember. The police interviewed the dealer who had sold me the item. He told them where he had purchased it. Eventually they settled the blame on an antique runner who was known to them and brough him to trial at Northampton Crown Court.

I was a witness for the prosecution and attended the Crown Court for the trial. This was my first and only experience of the law in action and a fascinating experience.

The first thing that happened was the choice of jurors. The candidates were paraded in front of the accused who agreed to them being used or not. One prospective juror turned out to be the accused maths teacher when he was at school. Needless to say he was rejected.

When I was called to be a witness I stood before the wigged judged and faced the jury. The barrister for the prosecution questioned me at great length and went on so long with irrelevant questions the judge told him to stop wasting time and get to the point. Basically all I could tell them was where and when I had purchased the clock, but the questioning went on for about twenty minutes.

After my time in front of the jury, I sat outside the court until I was given permission to go home. The dealer who had supplied me with the clock was questioned at great length, then I was allowed to go.

The accused was charged with stealing the clock but he admitted only to buying it from a third party. He would not disclose the third party's name because he feared for his safety. Justice was done and the accused was acquitted.

The dealer who sold me the clock was very honest and fair and refunded the money I had paid for it.

It was an interesting experience but one I don't particularly want to repeat!

Chapter Fourteen - In Conclusion

In conclusion, I can say I enjoyed my career as a Country Pharmacist. The pace of rural business gave me a chance to get to know my customers personally, which meant I could give them a better service. I have no regrets that I chose not to take promotion to a larger pharmacy when it was offered; that would have seperated me further from the public, a contact I enjoyed so much.

When I retired in 1995 I had practised pharmacy for over 40 years. I had seen a lot of changes but I enjoyed it all immensely. I went into pharmacy not knowing what to expect but landed in a profession that suited my temperament. I rapidly realised I was a people person and had found, by happy accident, a way of life that fitted me perfectly.

In retirement I continued my hobbies and added a new interest; I started creative writing more seriously. I had written since my school days getting poems printed in the School Magazine and selling a few articles, but I hadn't the time while working, to do much serious writing.

When I finished full time work I wrote and had published my first novel - The Faerie Stone, but the publisher closed his business unexpectedly and I received no royalties in spite of selling many copies and working hard to do that. After that unfortunate experience, I decided to set up my own publishing imprint and take complete control of my own work output. This was in 1997, long before Self- Publishing enjoyed the popularity and success it enjoys today. My second novel - The Tomatoes of Time - won the Best Novel category in the National Self-Publishing Awards for 1998.

Since that date I have written and published many titles including short stories and three song lyrics, which have been recorded by a folk singer.

Soon after retiring I stopped doing taxidermy work for the general public and wrote textbooks on the subject instead. Similarly with clocks, I wrote and published 'Care of the Longcase Clock' in 2007.

Sound advice given to any author is to write about what you know. I drew on my pharmacy experience for my five humorous fantasy novels, using my knowlege of chemists in the past to set the scenes.

The realisation that so much has altered in Pharmacy over the years has prompted me to share my experiences in these memoirs.

When I went into pharmacy the accent was on the preparation of medicines, now the Pharmacy degree is orientated more towards clinical pharmacy and is an M.Pharm. degree with four years study at university and one further year of practical training followed by another examination assessing the student's competence to practise.

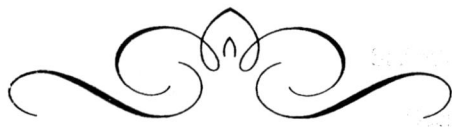

All available to order through book shops or direct from the publisher
www.rexmerchant.co.uk

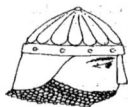

Published by
Rex Merchant

@ Norman Cottage